The Traveler's Compact Guide To Health, Illness & Safety

The Traveler's Compact Guide to Health, Illness, & Safety

Notices & How to Use this Guide

This guide is intended as a starting point for identifying some of the
important tasks required to prevent illness and injury that can occur
while traveling & vacationing. Information within this book cannot
replace evaluation by trained physicians to determine patient and
destination specific health risks associated with travel. Importantly,
it is impossible to diagnose & treat illness via a book. Only trained
health professionals can diagnose many disorders we have described.
This text can serve as a guide to begin a process of preventing and
initiating treatment of travel related illness and injury. Professional
medical care will be required for almost all disorders in this book.

Units of Measure in US vs. International/Metric System

Length	• 1 inch = 2.54 centimeters [cm] (*1 cm = 0.394 inches*)
	• 1 foot = 0. 305 meters (*1 meter = 3.281 feet*)
	• 1 mile = 1.61 kilometers (*1 kilometer = 0.621 miles*)
Volume[1]	• 1 ounce [oz] = 29.6 milliliters [ml] (*1 ml = 0.034 oz*)
	• 1 cup = 0.237 liters [L] (*1 L = 4.227 cups*)
	• 1 gallon = 3.785 L (*1 L = 0.264 gallons*)
Weight	• 1 ounce = 28.35 grams (*1 gram = 0.035 ounces*)
	• 1 pound = 0.454 kilograms [kg] (*1 kg = 2.205 pounds*)
Speed	10 miles per hour = 16.1 kilometers per hour
Temp.	Fahrenheit (F) to Celsius (C): $C = (F - 32) * 0.56$
	Celsius to Fahrenheit: $F = (1.8 * C) + 32$

[1] In the United Kingdom (UK), 1 UK ounce = 28.41 ml, 1 UK gallon
= 4.55 L

Contacts: The following is a list of websites and phone numbers for researching and assisting with details about international trips including document requirements, road conditions, health risks, health insurance, assisting victims of crime, medical evacuation, and contact for medical assistance while traveling internationally.

Air Ambulance & Health Insurance for citizens traveling abroad: www.travel.state.gov/travel/tips/brochures/brochures_1215 1-800-863-0312 or 941-536-2002.
American Society of Tropical Medicine and Hygiene (health risks): www.astmh.org
Association for Safe International Road Travel (road conditions): www.asirt.org (1-301-983-5252)
Center for Disease Control (country specific health risks and vaccine recommendations): wwwn.cdc.gov/travel/destinationList.aspx
Divers Alert Network: www.diversalertnetwork.org (see page 90) 1-919-684-4326 or 1-919-684-8111 or 1-800-326-3822
Embassy/Consulate (passport, visas, country specific requirements): www.usembassy.gov **or** www.travel.state.gov/passport/passport_1738
Health Insurance for International Travelers: http://www.travel.state.gov/travel/tips/brochures/brochures_1215
International Association for Medical Assistance to Travelers International English speaking physicians – (You must 1ˢᵗ join – free with requested donation. You will be sent book with international English speaking physicians/ facilities) www.iamat.org
*International Society of Travel Medicine (travel health warnings & list of U.S. & international travel clinics):*www.istm.org
Overseas Citizens Services (US citizen medical+ victim assistance): http://travel.state.gov/travel/about/who/who_1245 1-202-501-4444 or 1-888-407-4747
Public Health Agency Canada (travel medicine experts in Canada): www.phac-aspc.gc.ca/tmp-pmv
US Department of State (visas, passports, travel warnings) http://travel.state.gov **or** www.state.gov/countries/
World Health Organization (country specific health risks): www.who.int/countries/en/

TRAVEL RISKS

Travelers should evaluate the risk of illness, injury and availability of medical care prior to their trip. While diseases and travel risks are often specific to the destination, several generalities can be made:

5 to 8% traveling to developed countries will become ill or injured.
Nearly 2/3 traveling to under-developed countries will become ill.
The most common travel illnesses are diarrhea & respiratory diseases.
Trauma is the #1 cause of death in younger travelers.
Cardiovascular disease is the #1 cause of death in older travelers.
Most travel illness & injury can be prevented with proper preparation.

PREPARATION

Prior to embarking on a trip, travelers should consider their personal state of health and the specific risks associated with the mode of travel and with their travel destination. Consider the following issues 6-8 weeks prior to leaving on your trip.

Country Specific Political Risks: The U.S. State Department has information regarding the political stability and information regarding health conditions, crime, security, and entry requirements for every country. (http://travel.state.gov/travel/cis_pa_tw/cis/cis_1765.html). Travel warnings and travel alerts are also posted for each specific country at this site and the Consular Affairs home page. (http://travel.state.gov) Alternately, the Overseas Citizens Services (1-888-407-4747 OR 1-202-501-4444) can answer questions regarding the safety of travel to particular regions of the world. Note: the toll free 888 number may not be accessible from overseas locations.

      If you are traveling to countries with high political, health, or crime risks, register with the US Department of State. (https://travelregistration.state.gov.) This will allow U.S. personnel to contact and assist you in case an emergency or crisis arises at your travel destination. This can be accomplished on line at (https://travelregistration.state.gov/ibrs/ui/).

Visas & Passports for US citizens: A *passport* is needed to identify yourself as a U.S. citizen for entering & leaving the US, and while in other countries. It can take 4-6 weeks to obtain a passport from the US government. New passport applications require an in-person visit to one of 9000 passport offices. See the US State Department website (http://travel.state.gov/passport/passport_1738) for these sites, the application and fee schedule. Other requirements include a valid photo identification, proof of US citizenship and 2 regulation photos (2 X 2 inches). Passport renewals can be completed by mail if you have an undamaged current passport, you received a passport within the prior 15 years, you were > 16 years old when your passport was 1st issued, & you still have the same name or can document a name change. After obtaining your passport, make 2 photocopies that show the passport number and the date and location of issue. Keep one copy with a trusted person residing at home and take a second copy with you on your trip (kept separate from your original documents). **(United Kingdom**: See www.ips.gov.uk/passport/travel.asp for recommendations.)

A *visa* is issued by your destination country. The question of whether you need a visa to travel to another country is decided by each country. To determine if a visa is required, contact your country's (US or UK) Embassy or Consulate of the country you plan to visit. If you are visiting several countries, you will have to apply to each country individually for a visa. Obtaining a visa can take an additional 2-3 months after you have your passport. *Expedited Passports & Visas*: In the US, expedited passports can be obtained in 2 weeks by contacting the National Passport Information Center (www.travel.state.gov/passport/get/first/first_831) or by calling 1-877-487-2778. This US State Department website describes what is needed to expedite the application. Alternately, multiple passport and visa service companies can expedite this process for a fee.

Lost or stolen passports: If your passport is lost or stolen overseas, contact the nearest American embassy or consulate to obtain a temporary passport. You will be required to complete a new passport application, prove who you are, bring 4 passport sized photographs (2 inches by 2 inches), show police report (if theft), and pay for the application. Having a photocopy of your passport with the passport number and date/place of issue can expedite the process.

INSURANCES (Health, Rental Car, & Travel):

Health Insurance: Before traveling, check your current health insurance to determine if you are covered for emergencies that occur abroad. Medicare and Medicaid do not cover treatment while traveling. Make sure that your insurance will pay for emergency transport including medical evacuation and payment for an air ambulance. When choosing a travel insurance company, make sure that pre-existing conditions (including pregnancy if needed) are covered and that the insurance carrier is aware of what activities you will undertake. Separate insurance for scuba diving may be required. If needed, contact the Diver's Alert Network/DAN at 1-800-446-2671 or online (www.diversalertnetwork.org/insurance/index.asp). If you require travel health insurance or medical evacuation, the US Department of State lists companies that provide these services. (http://travel.state.gov/travel/tips/brochures/brochures_1215) Included on this list are companies that will help identify appropriate physicians and healthcare provides if needed (e.g. International Association for Medical Assistance to Travelers: www.iamat.org).

Generally, overseas medical care is paid for at the time of service. Upon return home, you will have to contact your health insurance carrier for reimbursement. To assist with this process, make sure you obtain complete copies of all treatment and charges.

Auto Insurance: Check with your credit card to determine if they provide collision-damage coverage for car rentals abroad. Most overseas car rental agencies provide auto insurance although the cost and coverage can vary greatly from country to country. If travelers are driving long distances, some experts recommend renting a car from a country with lower rental and insurance costs (e.g. Germany) before driving to a country with much higher costs (e.g. Italy, Ireland). International Driving Permits only verify your US driver license information in 10 different languages and have no legal validity on their own. They can be obtained from the National Auto Club or the American Automobile Association.

Travel Cancellation-Interruption Insurance: Multiple large insurers will provide trip cancellation, trip interruption due to illness or accidents, travel delays due to weather, terrorism, or other unanticipated reasons. No specific companies can be recommended.

Personal Safety: It is easy for criminals to take advantage of tourists who do not know the language or their travel environment. Many common steps can prevent you from becoming a crime victim.

Personal Safety Tips

Review crime risk for each country (State Dept. website, page 4).
Dress casually where appropriate and wear little or no jewelry.
Buy clothes/accessories to hide passport, credit cards, and money.
Travel light and keep medicines & documents in carry-on luggage.
Use traveler's checks and only 1-2 major credit cards, not cash.
If you carry a wallet, keep it in your front pocket.
Do not let anyone hear or see you dial with a telephone credit card.
Keep your purse/handbag strap on a shoulder with the bag in front.
Be wary of crowding/jostling as this is a common pickpocket ploy.
Do not discuss room number or travel plans where you can be heard.
Stay on 3rd to 5th floor to limit criminal access & allow fire rescue.
Always lock your hotel room (windows too). Place valuables in safe.
Keep your room neat so you will notice disturbed or missing items.
Do not invite strangers to your room.
Review fire safety, including exits & equipment, at your hotel.
Do not travel outside at night unless you are in a large "safe" city.
If you are out at night, stay in large groups and in crowded areas.
Never swim alone or at night.
Do not accept a ride from strangers.
Do not accept food or drinks (alcohol or otherwise) from strangers.
Avoid illegal drugs (2000 Americans are arrested abroad each year).
Do not sleep in your car (esp. at the roadside)

Personal Safety continued ....

Back up Plans & Itinerary: Prior to leaving on a trip, leave a copy of your itinerary with family or friends at home in case they need to contact you. Make 2 copies of your passport identification, all tickets, credit cards, driver's license (& international driving permit), and a copy of the serial numbers of your traveler's checks. Leave one copy of each with family or friends at home and secure the other copy separate from the originals when you travel.

Emergency Contact when traveling: Prior to traveling obtain the phone number and address of the US embassy/consulate for your destination(www.travel.state.gov/travel/cis_pa_tw/cis/cis_1765.html) Keep this information in a secure location while traveling. Another resource for assistance while abroad is the Overseas Citizens Services which can be contacted at the following telephone numbers. (1-888-407-4747 or 1- 202-647-5225)

Hostage-Hijacking Situations:

The US State Department (http://travel.state.gov) details the risk of kidnapping for specific countries. Several factors can diminish your chance of being taken hostage. Avoid countries with a high risk of kidnapping. The possibility of being kidnapped can be diminished by avoiding common target areas (i.e. where Americans congregate), limiting discussions with strangers, varying routines and routes, walking purposefully (not appearing lost) and blending in. If captured, experts recommend the following: do not let the hostages think you are trying to identify them or escape, be polite, smile, avoid discussing sensitive political topics, make casual eye contact but avoid prolonged eye contact, eat what your are given, and sleep & exercise when possible. Most hostages are eventually released. Be aware that most hostages who die are killed during rescue attempts. If 1 hostage is killed (and rescuers know this), the possibility of an imminent rescue attempt increases. At the first sign of any rescue attempt, immediately drop to the floor and avoid sudden movements. Follow all directions of any rescuers and expect to be temporarily restrained until the situation stabilizes. The US government's policy is to make no concessions including ransom, prisoner release, policy changes or other special consideration to groups or individuals who hold US citizens hostage. However, the US government will work with the host country to protect hostages and affect their release.

General Medical Health

A general medical exam is important prior to leaving on any major trip. For older patients, cardiovascular health is important, particularly if heavy physical exertion will take place. Blood pressure should be controlled and a cardiac evaluation (e.g. stress test) may be required to ensure you can handle the physical stress associated with a trip. Address all unresolved medical issues prior to any trip. Prior to travel, all routine vaccinations should be up to date.

Adult Routine (Standard) Vaccination Schedule[1]

Vaccine[2]	19-49 years	50-64 years	≥ 65 years
Td or Tdap	Td every 10 years (if < 65 years, give one Tdap)		
HPV	3 doses if female ≤ 26 years old given at time 0, then repeated 2 & 6 months later (if unvaccinated)		
MMR	1 or 2 doses	1 dose	
Varicella	A dose at time zero, then repeat in 4-8 weeks		
Influenza	If risk factors[3]	1 dose	
Pneumococcal	1 doses, repeated in 5 years[4]		1 dose
Hepatitis A	2 doses at time 0 and 6-18 months[5]		
Hepatitis B	3 doses at time 0, 1-2 months, then 4-6 months[5]		
Meningococcal	1 or more doses[6]		
Herpes Zoster			1 dose
Shaded	This dosing is recommended if additional risk present (e.g. underlying disease, job, lifestyle)		
Unshaded	Standard dosing if correct age and lack immunity (e.g. no prior infection or no vaccination)		

[1] If pregnant, HIV positive, diabetes, chronic heart/lung disease, alcoholism/liver/kidney disease, blood disorders or a weak immune system or health care worker, a different regimen may be needed.
[2] Td/Tdap – tetanus (T), diphtheria (d), acellular pertussis (ap), HPV – human papillomavirus, MMR – measles, mumps, rubella
[3] If diabetes, heart, lung (including asthma), kidney/liver/blood disease, or a weak immune or respiratory system.
[4] If diabetes, heart, lung (not asthma), kidney/liver/blood disease, weak immune system, cochlear implant, nursing home, native American and native Alaskan population
[5] If exposure to blood, persons with hepatitis, or travel to endemic areas. For other indications see www.cdc.gov.
[6] If no spleen function, 1st year college students living in dormitory, or travel to Mecca or endemic countries (e.g. sub-Saharan Africa)

Child & Adolescent Standard Immunizations

Those who have undergone vaccination series needed for school in United States are usually up to date with standard immunizations. See www.cdc.gov/vaccines/recs/schedules/ for recommendations.

Immunizations - Travel Vaccine Recommendations
Infectious Disease Society of America (See pregnancy, page 15)

Standard vaccines	A complete standard adult or child vaccination series is needed for all travelers. See page 9.
Japanese B Encephalitis (JE) IXIARO preferred if available & not contraindicated	Indicated if living > 1 mo in endemic/epidemic area during JE transmission season or traveling to rural farm areas where virus is found. (IXIARO) given as 2 doses, 28 days apart. It is not approved if < 17 years old. OR (Je-VAX) It is given on day 0, then repeated 7 and 30 days later. Not approved if < 1 year old.
Meningo-coccal (see page 111)	Indicated (10 days pre-travel) if visit endemic, epidemic area, pilgrimage to Saudi Arabia, college freshman, no spleen or immune deficient
Rabies	See page 54 for detail regarding rabies vaccine.
Tuberculosis (BCG)	BCG vaccine is generally only recommended for health care workers who have ongoing exposure to patients with resistant TB.
Typhoid (Typhim or Vivotif)	Vaccine (Typhim-shot, Vivotif-oral) is indicated if travel to small city or rural site that is endemic Vaccines are only 50-80% effective and must be given 2 weeks pre-travel.
Yellow Fever (YF-Vax)	Indicated if travel to endemic area or if required by a specific country. It must be given at least 10 days pre travel Do not give if < 9 months old.

Other vaccines may be required depending upon destination. Use travel expert to determine indications/contraindications.

Medications & Equipment

Keep a list of all medications with generic names, doses, and directions in safe location. Place medications securely within carry-on luggage. Consider obtaining and storing extra doses of important medications separately. Pack extra contact lenses, glasses, or necessary medical equipment (i.e. insulin syringes) & put together a first aid or medical kit appropriate for your destination. (See page 11)

Travel Medical Kit Contents

Depending upon a traveler's destination, a variety of items may be useful for preventing or treating minor disease and injury.

Personal Items & Equipment	
Contact lenses and glasses (plus extras), insulin syringes/needles	
Printed medical history and medical contact at home and travel site	
Medications & Remedies	
All medicines	All medicines require the original container with listed generic names and a note from the treating physician for all controlled and injectable medicines
1ˢᵗ Aid items	Bandages, gauze, ace wrap, tape, scissors
Allergic reaction	Topical hydrocortisone, diphenhydramine (*Benadryl*), Epinephrine (*Epi-Pen*) if history of severe allergic reactions
Blisters	Moleskin or sports tape
Cleansers	Antibacterial hand wipe or alcohol based hand cleanser
Cough medicine decongestant	Dextromethorphan (cough suppressant), guaifenesin (expectorant), pseudoephedrine or phenylephrine (decongestants)
Dehydration	Oral rehydration packets
Diarrhea	See pages 87-89
Fever	Acetaminophen[1]/*Tylenol,* ibuprofen/*Motrin*
Insect repellant	DEET based repellants
High altitude	See page 50 for options
Malaria	See page 99-101 for options
Motion sickness	Dimenhydrinate (*Dramamine*), meclizine (*Antivert*)
Pain relief	See fever above or any anti-inflammatory
Skin trauma	Topical antibiotic
Sleep aid	Melatonin, zolpidem (*Ambien*)
Sunscreen/sunburn	SPF 15 or greater sunscreen and aloe gel
Vomiting	Ondansetron (*Zofran*), phenergan
Water purification	Water purification tablets (e.g. chlorine dioxide, chlorine, iodine)

[1] acetaminophen is called paracetamol in the United Kingdom

Food and Water

Water in under developed countries can be contaminated with human and animal waste, viruses, parasites, and bacteria, decaying vegetation, pollutants, or from minerals or soil. Normal appearance and taste are NOT reliable methods for determining contamination. Even in the United States, almost none of the surface water is drinkable without treatment. Sources of safe food and water and methods for risk reduction are listed (Table: Safety of Food & Water, Table: Methods for Sterilizing Water).

Food & Water that is Safe/Unsafe to Eat or Drink

Generally Safe *(Listed Food & Beverages are usually but not always safe)*	• Commercially bottled water, soft drinks, fruit juices, or alcoholic drinks only if they are unopened. See page 13 for water sterilization techniques. • Hot tea and heated coffee (if water heated over time or if water was boiled) • Fruits and vegetables that you peeled are safer than those do not require peeling (be sure to wash surface before peeling). Beware that melons are often punctured and injected with water to increase market weight and sales price. • Hard boiled eggs served in intact shell • Meat and fish recently cooked with no pink areas (not re-warmed meat) • Milk and dairy products in Australia, Canada, Japan, United States, and Western Europe • Canned milk
Unsafe	• All surface water (streams, ponds, wells) • Anything poured into a glass or that has ice • Fruit and vegetables (all salads) that are already peeled or do not require peeling • Food that requires human handling or is only re-warmed (not re-cooked) prior to serving • Shellfish • Rare or raw meat, vegetables, fruit • Unpasteurized milk and milk products

Rapid Water Sterilization Techniques

Boiling	• Bring water to a boil, keep boiling for 1 minute (as a safety margin), then cover for several more minutes. This will kill almost all organisms causing gastrointestinal symptoms.
Chemicals (Halogens)	• <u>Chlorine dioxide</u> is superior to chlorine & iodine for killing viruses and Cryptosporidium. One *Aquamira* or *Micropur* tablet treats 1 Liter water. Wait 15-30 min. (40 min. to kill Cryptosporidium). • <u>Chlorine</u> kills bacteria and viruses while it is less effective vs. many parasites. Household bleach is 4-6% chlorine. Add 4 drops of 4-6% chlorine to 1 Liter water. Double the # of drops if water is cloudy or cold. Let stand for 30 minutes and use water if there is a slight chlorine smell. If no smell, repeat drops and let stand 15 minutes. • <u>Iodine</u> – kills bacteria, Giardia, and viruses but not Cryptosporidium. It is unsafe if pregnancy, or thyroid disease. Only use for short periods (< 1 month). Tablets and solutions are available and require different dosing based on concentration. A wait of 4 hours after mixing may be required.

Adjunctive & Alternative Water Cleansing Techniques

Adsorption	• Granular activated charcoal can be used to adsorb chemicals (e.g. after adding halogens).
Citrus (lime juice)	• Not rigorously studied (esp. against parasites) • Use only as a last resort, does not always work • Add 2 tablespoons (30 ml) to 1 Liter water
Filtration	• Filters remove large organisms but **do not** remove or kill viruses. Purifiers remove large organisms & add halogens (see chemicals) to kill viruses
Sediment-ation	• Letting water stand settles large particles in 3 hours & 90% of cysts (Cryptosporidium, Giardia) in 48 hours. Don't use this method alone.
Ultraviolet Light	• UV light (commercial pen lights) kills virtually all organisms. Water must be clear to work.

Pregnancy and Travel

Timing of travel: Several important issues arise when travelers are pregnant. An obstetrical evaluation should be performed to ensure that the traveler is healthy and has no pregnancy related or underlying medical disorders that might impact the mother or fetus. According to the American College of Obstetrics and Gynecology (ACOG), the safest time to travel is during mid-pregnancy or between 14-28 weeks. Morning sickness has usually resolved by then and the enlarging uterus does not hamper movement as much as it does during the last trimester (beyond 28 weeks). The quickest method of travel is the best so that any medical problem arising during travel can be handled quickly after arriving at destination.

Travel modes: When traveling by car, the ACOG recommends wearing a shoulder belt and a lap belt **below** the uterus and on the hip bones. The ACOG also recommends keeping air bags turned on. Travel by air is almost always safe during pregnancy and most airlines allow pregnant women to travel until they are 35 weeks pregnant if international travel and 36 weeks pregnant if travelling within the United States and Canada (1 month prior to their due date). Pregnant women should bring documentation of their due date or stage of pregnancy in addition to their health records, visa, passport, and immunization records regardless of their mode of travel. If possible, identify and investigate available options for medical care during travel and at the destination prior to travel. Ensure that your health insurance will cover pregnancy related complications during travel.

Several physiologic changes impact the pregnant traveler. Total blood volume increases 40-50% during a normal pregnancy causing a normal anemia or a dilution of hemoglobin (the molecule carrying oxygen). To compensate, the respiratory center increases the depth of breathing which leads to a feeling of shortness of breath during the last half of pregnancy. These changes will limit exercise capacity and require frequent rests if prolonged walking or climbing occur. An enlarging uterus obstructs urinary flow and leads to an increased risk of urine infections. To offset this risk, pregnancy women should stay hydrated and not delay voiding when they have to urinate.

Physiologic changes continued: Weight gain & redistribution, and relaxation of ligaments alter walking and climbing which places pregnant women at risk for muscle/joint pain, and falling. Blood clots within the legs and lungs may occur (esp. during the last trimester-3months). Stay hydrated & mobile to minimize this risk.
Vaccines: All women require appropriate vaccinations **before** pregnancy if possible. The US Food and Drug Administration categorizes all vaccines except human papilloma virus as category C meaning their safety is uncertain, animal studies may show an adverse effect, no well controlled human studies exist, and potential benefits may warrant use in pregnancy despite potential risks. In general, inactivated vaccines are considered safe and tetanus, diphtheria, and influenza vaccines are routinely given in pregnancy. Live vaccines are generally NOT used in pregnancy (Table).

Pregnancy Immunizations[1]

Inactivated or Polysaccharide or Recombinant	
Cholera toxin B	NOT recommended, Some use if very high risk
Hepatitis A and B	Recommended if indicated
Influenza	Recommended after 12-14th week pregnancy
Japanese encephalitis	Data unavailable. Weigh risk of vaccine against risk of disease.
Meningococcal	Recommended for high risk exposures
Pneumococcal	Use only if high risk pregnancy (e.g. no spleen)
Polio (IPV)	Recommended if indicated
Rabies	Recommended post-exposure if indicated
Tetanusdiphtheria	Recommended if indicated
Typhoid Vi	Use only if clearly indicated
Live attenuated virus	
Cholera	Do not use live attenuated oral cholera vaccine.
Measles-mumps-rubella	Do not give. If exposed to diseases may receive immune globulin to prevent disease.
Typhoid Ty21a	Do not give.
Varicella	Do not give. If exposed to disease, may receive varicella immune globulin to prevent disease if not immune by blood tests or by history.
Yellow fever	Only consider if exposure unavoidable

[1] See specific disease & vaccination section (page 9-10 for detail).

Pregnancy & Travel

Malaria prophylaxis and treatment: Travel to areas of the world with active malaria can be unsafe and requires extra precautions.
DEET insect repellants are generally safe and it is recommended that they may be used sparingly in pregnancy. Mefloquine, chloroquine, (atovaquone plus proguanil) are antimalarial agents that are usually avoided in the first 3 months of pregnancy. If travel to high malaria risk areas, some experts administer mefloquine in the 1st 3 months of pregnancy. If indicated for treatment or prophylaxis, travel medicine, and infectious disease experts will recommend one of these agents after the 1st 3 months of pregnancy. Primaquine & doxycycline are avoided during all stages of pregnancy.

Infants and Children

Infants under 2 years or < 15 kilograms have an increased risk of acquiring disease compared to older children and adults when traveling to under developed countries. They are incompletely immunized, have weaker immune systems, are less hygienic, and may not be able to receive vaccinations or other medications that can protect them. Parents should consider this risk when traveling.
Vaccination: In addition to standard vaccines (page 10), a medical visit should be made 6 weeks prior to travel to determine if additional vaccines are indicated. Vaccination can be undertaken for yellow fever at 9 months old, typhoid (2-6 years for VICPS, > 6 years for oral live attenuated), meningococcal [ACYW-135] (2 years), Japanese encephalitis (1 year), rabies (birth), and early hepatitis A (1-2 years). If any of these vaccines are indicated, they should be initiated 4-6 weeks prior to travel.
Malaria: Children < 5 years are the most vulnerable population and are more likely to die from malaria compared to older children and adults. Chloroquine is used for travel to chloroquine sensitive areas (Caribbean, Central America north of Panama, Middle East), while mefloquine (*Lariam*) is used in chloroquine resistant areas. Mefloquine is not used if seizures, psychiatric illness, or heart rhythm abnormalities are present. Instead doxycycline or (atovaquone plus proguanil) are used. If symptoms of malaria develop and medical care is unavailable, pyrimethamine-sulfadoxine (*Fansidar*) can be started for those older than 2 months who are not G6PD deficient.

International Phone Service & Cellphones/World Phones

Cell phones used in the North and South America may not work when taken to Europe, Africa and Asia. There are two competing network technologies, CDMA (Code Division Multiple Access) and GSM (Global System for Mobile Communication). CDMA phones are only available in the United States and parts of Asia and thus, usually cannot be used internationally. GSM networks are common internationally.

In North and South America, GSM networks use frequencies of 850 or 1900 while in Europe and Asia these frequencies are 900 or 1800. There are rare phones (quad-band phones) that work with all four bands/frequencies. In general, phones that work with at least 3 of these frequencies can be used in all countries and are called "World Phones". Some cell phone companies do not offer international cell phone service and their phones may be "locked" such that you will not be able to add a SIM (subscriber information module) card to a phone with a new cell phone number and new network. There are several options for obtaining cell phone service internationally.

First, if you have a CDMA phone, you will not be able to use it internationally. If you have a GSM phone, contact your current cell phone service to determine if your phone is locked (i.e. no SIM card can be added), if it works with the GSM standard of the country to which you are traveling, and what charges will accrue using your current cell phone carrier (if it is available internationally).

Option 1: Rent or purchase an unlocked cell phone that works on the GSM network of the country to which you are traveling. A SIM card that works at your destination also will be needed.

Option 2: Use your current GSM cell phone if it is compatible with the standard at your destination, it can be unlocked, and you have a cell phone plan that allows for international roaming charges. A SIM card will be required with a new cell phone number and compatibility with international networks. This option may be expensive and might be the best option if few calls are made (i.e. only emergency calls)

Preparation Checklist Prior to Travel

	Access the state department websites to assess the political, climate, and safety risks associated with particular countries.
	Register with the US State Department and give your itinerary to trusted person in the United States (or in your home country).
	Review & follow personal safety tips (pages 7-8).
	Obtain travel health insurance and car insurance (if needed).
	Undergo general medical exam to ensure you can travel.
	Undergo travel medicine or infectious disease expert evaluation if traveling to non-industrialized country.
	Keep list of prescription medications (generic names) in a secure location. If possible, keep back up prescription for each medication you take in separate locations.
	Undergo basic vaccinations (e.g. tetanus, influenza).
	Add exotic vaccinations (e.g. yellow fever) if traveling to sites with specific risk for diseases that can be prevented.
	Protect yourself against food and water borne illness.
	Protect yourself from mosquito borne illness (e.g. malaria).
	Understand and prepare for your destination climate & altitude.
	Put together a medical or 1st aid packet appropriate for your travel destination. (See page 11)

AIRLINES and ILLNESS

Any emergency or illness that occurs on the ground can also occur in the air. Between 1 in 14,000 and 1 in 40,000 passengers develop a medical emergency during flight with half requiring a visit to an emergency department and 10% requiring hospital admission. Deaths occur in 1 in 1 million passengers with 75% due to heart disease or known medical problems.

The most common in-flight emergencies are blackouts, trauma (usually minor), abdomen pain/vomiting, and breathing difficulties. When an in-flight medical emergency occurs, the crew often asks for on-board medical personnel (physicians, nurses, paramedics) to assist. Many airlines have in-flight medical consultation by ground based physicians. The Federal Aviation Administration mandates that airplanes with a maximum payload capacity > 7,500 pounds and one flight attendant carry one automated external defibrillator and at least one enhanced Emergency Medical Kit (below). Depending upon the number of passenger seats, 1 to 4 First Aid Kits are carried.

Good Samaritan Laws: The1998 Aviation Medical Assistance Act limits the US Federal and State liability for individuals & airlines providing a medical response to in-flight emergencies unless "the individual, while rendering the assistance, is guilty of gross negligence or willful misconduct". Canada and the United Kingdom have similar laws protecting Good Samaritans. For other countries, laws where the airline is based are in effect. Australian law mandates that you have a duty to help ill passengers.

Standard Airline First Aid Kit

Contents	Number
Adhesive bandage compresses (1 inch)	16
Antiseptic swabs	20
Ammonia inhalants	10
Bandage compresses (4 inches)	8
Triangular bandage compresses (40 inches)	5
Arm splint, leg splint (non-inflatable)	1 each
Roller bandage (4 inches)	4
Adhesive tape (1 inch)	2
Bandage scissors	1

Standard Airline Emergency Medical Kits[1]

Type & Purpose	Contents and (Number of Doses Stocked or Pieces of Equipment)
Protection	• Non-permeable gloves (1 pair)
Diagnosis	• Blood pressure cuff (1) • Stethoscope (1)
Airway devices	• Oropharyngeal airways to keep airway open: 1 pediatric, 1 small adult, 1 large adult
Intravenous (IV) Set up & Materials for Administering IV Medications	• Tubing (1) with Y connectors (2) • Alcohol sponges (2) • Roll of 1 inch adhesive tape (1) • Tape scissors (1) • Tourniquet (1) • Saline bag with 500 ml (1) • Needles: 18 gauge (2), 20 gauge (2), 22 gauge (2) • Syringes: 5 ml (1), 10 ml (2)
Analgesics	• Acetaminophen, 325 mg (4) • Aspirin, 325 mg (4)
Allergy & Wheezing	• Diphenhydramine (*Benadryl*), 25 mg (4) • Diphenhydramine IV, 50 mg (2) • Metered dose inhaler (1) • See epinephrine intramuscular below
Heart Disease	• Nitroglycerin tablets 0.4 mg (10) • Aspirin (see analgesic above)
Hypoglycemia (low blood sugar)	• Dextrose, 50%/50 ml IV (1)
Resuscitation Drugs	• Atropine 0.5 mg – 5 ml (2) • Epinephrine for intramuscular injection 1:1,000 – 1 ml (2) • Epinephrine for intravenous injection 1:10,000 – 2 ml (2) • Lidocaine 100 mg in 5 ml (2)

[1] ml – milliliter, mg - milligram

Anesthesiology 2008; 108: 749-755.

Oxygen, Altitude, & Cabin Air: Traveling in airplanes poses several risks to travelers. Most airlines have a cruising altitude between 18,000 and 40,000 feet and cabin pressure is maintained between 5,000 - 8,000 feet. For healthy people, this altitude causes slight hypoxia (low blood oxygen) that is inconsequential. People with chronic lung disease, cystic fibrosis, or other serious heart or lung problems may develop difficulty breathing or chest pain while flying. If you have underlying lung disease, have your physician determine if air travel is safe and whether or not supplemental in flight oxygen will be needed. If supplemental oxygen is required, contact your airline one week in advance to arrange its use during your flight.

Cabin air within airplanes comes from cold dry outside air that is heated and compressed before being circulated. A catalytic converter is used to remove ozone and a charcoal filter removes organic compounds such as fuel vapors. Commercial aircraft that are < 15-20 years old re-circulate up to 50% of air in the cabin mixed with outside air. More modern airplanes pass air through high efficiency particular air (HEPA) filters which capture almost all bacteria, fungi, and larger viruses. Humidity can be as low as 10% contributing to dry eyes, a dry & irritated respiratory tract, dehydration, and wheezing in patients with lung disease. Avoiding alcohol, caffeine, saline nasal and eye drops, and maintaining hydration during air flight can limit these effects. Patients with asthma or chronic obstructive lung disease should keep their inhalant(s) in carry-on luggage in case wheezing develops.

Pressure Related Ear & Sinus Disease (Barotrauma): The middle ear is connected to the back of the mouth via the Eustachian tubes and the sinuses are connected to the nasal cavity via ostia or small openings. Upper respiratory infections including colds, sinusitis and middle ear infections can block these openings. During flight, pressure changes, cause the gases within the sinuses and middle ear to expand by as much as 25% leading to trauma (barotrauma), bleeding, and intense pain if their openings are blocked. One small study found that oral pseudoephedrine 120 mg given 30 minutes before take-off decreased ear pain in adults with a history of recurrent ear pain during flight. A similar study found that pseudoephedrine was NOT effective in children.

Blood Clots (Pulmonary Embolism & Deep Venous Thrombosis):
Blood clots or thromboemboli can develop within the legs during
prolonged air travel (esp. if > 6-8 hours). The most serious
complication of clots within the deep veins of the leg (deep venous
thrombi) occur when clots travel to the lungs and cause low blood
pressure (hypotension), low blood oxygen (hypoxia), and potentially
death. Dehydration and immobility contribute to their development.
Other risk factors include inherited or acquired clotting disorders,
cancer, pregnancy, leg trauma, cardiovascular disease, use of
estrogens, recent surgery and possibly tobacco use, obesity, and
varicose veins. Staying hydrated during travel and frequent
stretching are recommended to prevent clots. Other options for
decreasing your risk of developing clots might include support
stockings, aspirin or injection of low molecular weight heparin.

  Any leg pain, swelling or redness that occurs during or after
a recent air flight requires a medical evaluation and preferably a
Doppler ultrasound to exclude a clot. If a clot has traveled to the
lungs (i.e. pulmonary embolism), a myriad of symptoms can develop.
These include (but are not limited to) chest pain, shortness of breath,
cough, or lightheadedness (blacking out). Immediate medical
attention is required if there is any suspicion of blood clots that have
traveled to the lungs.

Jet Lag: During jet lag, a change in time zones causes the daily body
rhythms and the internal drive for sleep and wakefulness to be out of
sync with the new environment. Symptoms of poor sleep, fatigue,
headaches, GI upset, and irritability can last for days. Symptoms are
worse if $\geq$ 3 time zones are crossed and with eastward flights. Jet lag
can be lessened by staying hydrated, limiting alcohol & caffeine,
breaking long trips with a stop-over, and increased early exposure to
sunlight at the travel destination. For adults, a 2 to 5 milligram dose
of melatonin taken at bedtime for 2 to 4 days after arrival can
decrease daytime sleepiness and help reset the biological clock.
Zolpidem (*Ambien*) has been shown to improve sleep and decrease
jet lag symptoms in adults flying eastward if given as 10 mg during
the flight and continued each night for 4 days. Importantly, these
drugs and other sleep promoting agents have multiple potential side
effects and their use should be discussed with your physician.

Diving & Airlines: Decompression sickness (the bends) can be precipitated by flying soon after diving. See pages 90-94 for details. For this reason, the Federal Aviation Administration recommends that divers should not fly for at least 24 hours after diving. The Divers Alert Network recommends a minimum of 12 hours before flying for a single No Decompression Dive and a minimum of 18 hours before flying for multiple <u>No Compression Limit Dives</u>. For dives requiring Decompression Stops, a longer preflight surface interval before flying is required. Importantly, a diver who needs to be medically evacuated by air requires the cabin pressure to be maintained at sea level.

Children: The Federal Aviation Administration (FAA) does not mandate the use of child safety seats on airplanes. The FAA's decision was based on their estimation that a mandate would cause more families to travel by car which statistically is much riskier than flying. Both the American Academy of Pediatrics and the FAA recommend using a child restraint system (CRS) that is rear facing for infants who are < 1 year old and < 20 pounds. A forward facing CRS is recommended for infants and children > 1 year old who weight 20-40 pounds. Those who weight > 40 pounds can be secured in an aircraft seat belt.

Pregnancy & Air Flight: The American College of Obstetricians and Gynecologists state that healthy pregnant women without complications can travel internationally up until their 35th week of pregnancy and domestically up to 36 weeks. The best time to travel is mid pregnancy between the 14th and 28th weeks since early travel may exacerbate morning sickness and mobility is limited in late pregnancy. Women with either medical or obstetric complications including hypertension, diabetes with poor glucose control, sickle cell disease, placental abnormalities, or risk factors for premature labor should avoid air travel.

In addition to their passport, visa, and immunization record, pregnant women should bring a letter from their doctor with their due date. This letter or other documentation of pregnancy status and due date may be required for travel.

CRUISE SHIPS

Overview: Guidelines exist for health care on cruise ships that mandate disease sanitation, disease surveillance, and varying degrees of healthcare depending upon the size, age, and ship's destination.. Cruise lines operating in the US or that belong to the International Council for Cruise Lines meet or exceed guidelines established by the American College of Emergency Physicians. Ships are required to have medical staff available 24 hours/day, 1 exam room, 1 critical care bed per ship, and 1 inpatient bed for every 1000 passengers. Advanced life support equipment and medications, and basic X-rays and available simple laboratory tests are mandated. While respiratory diseases and injuries are the most common reasons for visiting a ships infirmary, any disease occurring on land can occur on a cruise ship. Patients ≥ 65 years old accounted for more than half of all infirmary visits in one study. (Table)

Break Down of Illness/Injury Occurring on Cruise Ships

Respiratory disorders (infections and wheezing)	29%
Injuries (10% of injuries were fractures)	18%
Nervous system or sensory organ diseases	9%
Abdominal disease (vomiting, diarrhea, abdomen pain)	9%
Muscular & Skin disorders, arthritis (not injury related)	5%
Cardiac, vascular , circulatory disorders	3%
Genital, urinary disorders	3%
Mental illness, cancer, diabetes, other illness	24%

Motion (Sea) Sickness: Motion sickness occurs when the brain receives conflicting input from motion sensors in the body: the eyes, the inner ear, and position sensors within the body surface & joints (proprioceptors). Symptoms include nausea, vomiting, sweating, and a spinning sensation (vertigo). Treatment options include antihistamines (diphenhydramine/*Benadryl,* meclizine/*Antivert*), anticholinergics (scopolamine), vomiting medicines (dimenhydrinate /*Dramamine*), promethazine/*Phenergan* and ondansetron/*Zofran*). Suitability of these drugs requires discussion with your doctor.

Gastrointestinal Illness: The most common infective agent causing vomiting & diarrhea on ships has been the norovirus due to the low dose of virus required to cause infection, its ability to survive cleaning, and its easy transmissibility between passengers. In some outbreaks > 30% of all passengers can become infected.

Symptoms of norovirus include sudden onset of vomiting and diarrhea. Fever is **un**common and diarrhea usually does not contain blood. Dehydration, low potassium, and renal insufficiency can occur esp. in the elderly or those with underlying disease. Treatment includes replenishing fluids with balanced electrolyte solutions (e.g. *Pedialyte, Ricelyte, Gatorade, Powerade*). Medications (promethazine [*Phenergan*] or ondansetron [*Zofran*]) may limit vomiting and aid in fluid and electrolyte replacement. Ondansetron can be use in infants while promethazine should not be used in those ≤ 2 to 5 years old. Intravenous fluids may be required for those who become extremely dehydrated. Antibiotics are of no use in norovirus infection. Other types of infectious diarrhea occurring on ships include *Staphylococcus aureus* (onset < 6 hours from ingestion) and bacteria and parasites including Salmonella, E. coli, Shigella, Vibrio, Clostridium, & Cyclospora. Invasive bacteria can cause fever and bloody diarrhea. Antimicrobials may be used for bacteria & parasites.

Respiratory Infections: While any respiratory tract virus can easily be transmitted between passengers, two important diseases causing outbreaks on cruise ships include influenza & Legionnaires' disease. While usually a winter disease, influenza can occur at any time of year in the tropics. Symptoms include fever, muscle aches, cough, and sore throat. Influenza often resolves on its own except in those who are older or have underlying lung or heart disease. A secondary bacterial pneumonia can occur on top of this virus and can be deadly. (See influenza and respiratory infections, page 115-117)

Legionnaires' disease is due to a bacteria that grows in warm stagnant freshwater (e.g. pool spa) and outbreaks have been reported on cruise ships. Young, healthy victims develop an influenza-like illness with no pneumonia. The elderly and those with underlying heart and lung disease can develop a deadly pneumonia. Patients with pneumonia develop cough, fever, chills, chest pain and shortness of breath. Vomiting, diarrhea, headache, muscle aches, and an altered mental status can occur. Treatment consists of oxygen, fluids, blood pressure and cardiac support and intravenous antibiotics from the macrolide class of antibiotics (erythromycin, clarithromycin, azithromycin) or doxycycline. Care in an intensive care unit is often required. (See Legionnaires' disease, page 117)

ROAD (CAR & BUS) SAFETY

Traffic accidents are the leading cause of death in young travelers. In non-industrialized countries, mortality from car accidents is 20 to 80 times higher than in industrialized countries. Even in industrialized countries, the risk of injury or death from traffic accidents can be high due to unfamiliarity with road regulations, road conditions, and poor emergency medical systems.

The Association for Safe International Road Travel maintains a database of information regarding specific road safety information for each country. Before traveling, access this information at (www.asirt.org). While direct use of this website requires a contribution, you can receive free information regarding a particular country by sending an inquiry to the following email: asirt@asirt.org. The Road Safety Tips table details important safety tips to ensure you are not injured either as a passenger or pedestrian.

Road Safety Tips

Learn the local road rules, laws, and "culture". Access the website www.asirt.org prior to deciding to drive on your own.
Avoid traveling at night (esp. in countries with poor roads, poor safety records, or dangerous terrain).
Avoid cars, taxis, or buses that are dangerous appearing (e.g. top heavy) or that lack safety equipment (e.g. seat belts).
If a taxi or bus driver is driving dangerously or appears to be intoxicated, immediately exit the vehicle.
Wear seat belts at all times and only ride in taxis or cars with adequate occupant restraints.
Make sure that any vehicle you are driving has adequate tires, brakes, lighting, and windshield wipers.
If you are not used to driving on the opposite side of the road, undergo training prior to performing this task.
Avoid 2 wheeled transportation (e.g. motorcycle, scooter). If you choose to travel via this method, use a helmet at all times.
Do not use a cell phone or attempt to read any materials including a map while driving.
While walking wear bright clothes (reflective clothes at night), and stay on designated walkways (lit areas at night).
Keep cell phone, 1st aid kit, emergency contact with you always.
Do no hitchhike and do not pick up hitchhikers.

OVERVIEW

Certain diseases are associated with travel to specific regions around the world. Travelers should be aware of the common diseases causing illness for their destination. The GeoSentinel Global Surveillance Network of the International Society of Travel Medicine and the Centers for Disease Control has detailed the most common complaints and diseases in traveler's who return from a trip and <u>present to travel medicine clinics</u>.

The most common overall illness are detailed below with a breakdown of most common illness by region listed on pages 31, 35, 36, 39, 41, 46. Diseases causing fever is detailed page 96.

Illness in Returning Travelers – All Regions

Diagnosis or Illness[1]	% All Cases
Fever Related Illness **Viral illness** or no cause of illness found, Malaria, Dengue, Mononucleosis, Rickettsia, Salmonella (typhoid or typhoid related)	23%
Acute Diarrhea **Parasite** (Giardia or amoeba), Bacterial (Campylobacter, Shigella, Salmonella – nontyphoid)	22%
Skin Disorders & Rashes **Insect bite**, Cutaneous larval migrans, Skin abscess, Fungal, Leishmaniasis, Myiasis, Swimmer's itch, impetigo, Mites/scabies	17%
Chronic Diarrhea	11%
Abdominal Disease without Diarrhea Intestinal **nematode**/worms (Strongyloides, Ascaris), Gastritis or peptic ulcer, Hepatitis	8%
Respiratory Disease	8%
Genitourinary Disease	4%
Exacerbation of Chronic Disease already present, Neurologic Disease or Injury	2% each
Cardiovascular Disease, Obstetric/Gynecologic, Eye, Dental Disease	≤ 1% each

[1] Subsets under major diagnoses are listed in order of frequency with the most common diagnoses overall listed in bold.

AFRICA (NORTH) TRAVELER

Algeria	Egypt	Madeira Isle(s)	Tunisia
Canary Isle(s)	Libya	Morocco	Western Sahara

Food/Waterborne Infections & Sanitation[1]
Clean water and sanitation are poor and unreliable in most regions. Water and food-borne precautions should be maintained throughout travel.

Diarrhea caused by bacteria, parasites, and viruses is common even in many large cities.

Hepatitis A, B, and *C* are endemic to many areas with up to 18% living in Egypt infected with hepatitis C. Hepatitis A and B vaccination is recommended.

Mosquito, Tick, & Fly Flea borne Illness[1]
Dengue has been reported but is uncommon in North Africa.

Leishmaniasis (skin and organ) is carried by sand flies and occurs in this region.

Malaria is uncommon in most of North Africa although it is found in parts of Algeria and Egypt. Prophylaxis is required if traveling to malaria endemic regions within these countries. Chloroquine resistance is uncommon. (See Malaria, page 99-101)

Yellow fever is uncommon and vaccination is usually not recommended.

Mediterranean spotted fever (dog ticks), relapsing fever (ticks, lice) and murine typhus (fleas), and viral hemorrhagic fevers are present.

Other Infectious Risks[1]
Other important or common diseases include Brucellosis (unpasteurized milk), echinococcus (esp. Tunisia), HIV, leptospirosis, polio, schistosomiasis (esp. Nile delta), tuberculosis, worms (hookworms, roundworms, whipworms)

[1] Disease lists are NOT all inclusive and leave out many common and unique diseases. See wwwn.cdc.gov/travel/destinationList.aspx for detail about vaccine and medicine prophylaxis recommendations.

AFRICA (SUB-SAHARAN) TRAVELER

Countries that Comprise Sub-Saharan Africa

Central Africa		South Africa	
Angola	Democrat Rep	Botswana	South Africa
Cameroon	Congo (Zaire)	Lesotho	Swaziland
Central African Republic	Equatorial Guinea	Namibia	Zimbabwe
Chad	Gabon		
Congo	Sudan		
	Zambia		

West Africa		East Africa	
Benin	Mali	Burundi	Mayotte
Burkina Faso	Mauritania	Comoros	Mozambique
Cape Verde	Niger	Djibouti	Reunion
Cote d'Ivoire	Saint Helena	Eritria	Rwanda
(Ivory Coast)	Sao Tome and	Ethiopia	Seychelles
Gambia	Principe	Kenya	Somalia
Ghana	Senegal	Madagascar	Tanzania
Guinea	Sierra Leone	Malawi	Uganda
Guinea-Bissau	Togo	Mauritius	
Liberia			

Food/Waterborne Infections & Sanitation[1]

Clean water and sanitation are unavailable or poor in most regions. Water and food-borne precautions should be maintained throughout travel.

Diarrhea caused by bacteria, parasites, and viruses is common even in many large cities. *Cholera* is especially common in health care and refugee camp workers (esp. West & Central Africa). Use of a cholera vaccine is recommended in this population. *Typhoid fever* is common and pre-travel vaccination is generally recommended if traveling to this region.

Hepatitis A, B, and *C* are common in most of Sub-Saharan Africa. Up to 10% of some populations carry hepatitis B. All travelers should receive vaccination against hepatitis A and B prior to travel.

Mosquito, Tick, Fly & Flea borne Illness[1]

African sleeping sickness (Trypanosomiasis) is present in Central and East Africa and those who visit game parks are most at risk. Importantly, insect repellants are not uniformly effective in preventing bites from the carrier (tsetse fly).

Dengue is uncommon in most areas although the mosquito that transmits this disease is present in many Sub-Saharan countries.

Leishmaniasis (skin and organ) is carried by sand flies and occurs in this region.

Malaria is common throughout Sub-Saharan Africa with outbreaks most common after the rainy season. Prophylaxis is required if traveling to most Sub-Saharan regions. Chloroquine resistance is common. (See Malaria, page 99-101)

Yellow fever has been recently reported in Angola, Cameroon, Gambia, Guinea, Kenya, Mali, Nigeria, Sudan, and Zaire. Certification of vaccination is required for travel to many Sub-Saharan countries.

African tick bite fever (esp. Southern African countries), murine typhus (flea), epidemic typhus (louse), filariasis, Onchocerciasis or river blindness (black fly), and viral hemorrhagic fevers are found here.

Other Infectious Risks[1]

Other important or common diseases include amebiasis, brucellosis (unpasteurized milk), HIV, Lassa fever, meningitis (vaccination is required with quadrivalent meningococcal vaccine pre-travel), plague (rodents), Q fever, rabies, schistosomiasis, tuberculosis, typhoid fever (esp. Congo), and worms (hookworms, roundworm, shipworms, Strongyloides).

[1] Disease lists are NOT all inclusive and leave out many common and unique diseases. See wwwn.cdc.gov/travel/destinationList.aspx for detail about vaccine and medicine prophylaxis recommendations.

Most Common Cause of Fever in Sub-Saharan Traveler

Diagnosis or Illness[1]	% of all cases
Malaria	62%
No Cause Found	28%
Rickettsia (e.g. typhus)	6%
Mononucleosis (Epstein Barr or cytomegalovirus)	1%
Salmonella typhi or *Salmonella paratyphi*	1%
Dengue	1%

Most Common Cause of Acute Diarrhea - Sub-Saharan Traveler

Diagnosis or Illness[1]	% of all cases
Viral illness or no cause found	40%
Parasite Giardia (18% of all diarrhea cases) Amoeba (14% of all diarrhea cases)	35%
Bacterial (*E.coli* also common) Campylobacter (7% of all diarrhea) Shigella (5% of all diarrhea) Non-typhoidal salmonella (3%)	25%

Most Common Skin Disorders in Sub-Saharan Traveler

Diagnosis or Illness[1]	% of all cases
Insect bite with/without other infection	19%
Skin abscess or impetigo, erysipelas	17%
Swimmer's itch (Schistosomiasis)	12%
Allergic reaction or allergic rash	11%
Cutaneous Larva Migrans	9%
Mycosis (fungal)	7%
Myiasis	4%
Leishmaniasis	1%
Mites (e.g. scabies)	1%

Most Common Gastrointestinal Disorders Without Diarrhea

Diagnosis or Illness[1]	% of all cases
Nematode/worms (Strongyloides, Ascaris)	31%
Gastritis or ulcer	9%
Hepatitis	8%

ASIA TRAVELER

Central (South) Asia		East Asia	
Afghanistan	India	China	Mongolia
Bangladesh	Maldives	Hong Kong	North Korea
Bhutan	Nepal	Japan	South Korea
British Indian	Pakistan	Macau	Taiwan
Ocean	Sri Lanka		

Southeast Asia			
Brunei	Cambodia	Laos	Singapore
Burma	East Timor	Malaysia	Thailand
(Myanmar)	Indonesia	Philippines	Vietnam

Central Asia (also called South Asia)

Food/Waterborne Infections & Sanitation – Central Asia[1]
Clean water and sanitation are poor. Water and food-borne precautions should be maintained throughout travel.

Diarrhea caused by bacteria, parasites, and viruses is common. Cholera is common in Bangladesh and India. Cysticercosis is prominent in India. Typhoid & paratyphoid fever, (resistant to common antibiotics) & amebic infection (with liver abscesses) occur.

Hepatitis A and *B* are common. Outbreaks of hepatitis E have also occurred.

Mosquito, Tick, & Fly Flea borne Illness – Central Asia[1]
Dengue occurs in most Central Asian countries.
Japanese encephalitis occurs in most lowland areas of Central Asia.
Leishmaniasis (skin and organ) is carried by sand flies and occurs in this region (esp. Afghanistan, Bangladesh, India, Nepal, Pakistan,
Malaria is found at altitudes below 2000 meters above sea level.
Yellow fever does not occur in Asia despite the presence of the mosquito vector (Aedes aeqypti). Other vector born infections include epidemic typhus (louse), filariasis (mosquito), murine typhus (flea), relapsing fever (tick), scrub typhus (chigger), and spotted fever (tick).

Other Infectious Risks - Central Asia[1]

Other important or common diseases include anthrax, avian influenza (bird flu), echinococcosis, plague, Q fever, tuberculosis,

---

East Asia

Food/Waterborne Infections & Sanitation – East Asia[1]

Clean water and sanitation are good and water is generally safe to drink in Hong Kong and Japan. Otherwise, water and food-borne precautions should be maintained throughout travel.

Diarrhea caused by bacteria, parasites, and viruses is common. Liver flukes are an important water born disease in this region. Brucellosis and cholera are found in most areas (except Japan). Schistosomiasis is especially common in the Yangtze River basin.

Hepatitis A and *B* are common (except in Japan).

Mosquito, Tick, & Fly Flea borne Illness – EastAsia[1]

Dengue has been found in China, Hong Kong, and Taiwan. *Leishmaniasis* (skin and organ) is uncommon in East Asia. *Japanese encephalitis* occurs in China, Japan, and areas of Korea. *Yellow fever* does not occur in Asia despite the presence of the mosquito vector (Aedes aeqypti). Other vector born infections include epidemic typhus (louse), filariasis (mosquito), murine typhus (flea), relapsing fever (tick), scrub typhus (chigger), and spotted fever (tick).

Other Infectious Risks East Asia[1]

Other important or common diseases include anthrax (rural, China, Mongolia), avian influenza (bird flu), echinococcosis (rural China, Mongolia), hantavirus (hemorrhagic fever with renal failure, esp. in China, South Korea), paragonimiasis (lung fluke), rabies, strongyloidiasis, tuberculosis,

---

[1] Disease lists are NOT all inclusive and leave out many common and unique diseases. See wwwn.cdc.gov/travel/destinationList.aspx for detail about vaccine and medicine prophylaxis recommendations.

Southeast Asia

Food/Waterborne Infections & Sanitation – Southeast Asia[1]

Clean water and sanitation are generally poor in Southeast Asia.

Diarrhea due to Campylobacter (often drug resistant) is especially prominent in Thailand although there are many other bacteria, viruses, and parasites that can cause diarrhea and liver abscesses. Cholera epidemics have been reported in multiple countries.

Hepatitis A and *B* are widespread and vaccination is recommended for most travelers. Hepatitis E is reported in Burma and Indonesia.

Mosquito, Tick, & Fly Flea borne Illness – Southeast Asia[1]

Dengue epidemics are common in this area.

Japanese encephalitis is widespread and occurs year round in tropical regions.

Leishmaniasis (skin and organ) is uncommon with Burma (Myanmar) reporting most cases.

Malaria is found throughout southeast Asia (except Brunei, Singapore) with Chloroquine and multidrug resistance reported.

Yellow fever does not occur in Asia despite the presence of the mosquito vector (Aedes aeqypti). Other vector born infections include filariasis (mosquito), murine typhus (flea), relapsing fever (tick), and scrub typhus (chigger).

Other Infectious Risks – Southeast Asia[1]

Other important or common diseases include anthrax (Burma), avian influenza (bird flu), cysticercosis (Indonesia) paragonimiasis (lung fluke), rabies, schistosomiasis, strongyloidiasis, tuberculosis,

[1] Disease lists are NOT all inclusive and leave out many common and unique diseases. See wwwn.cdc.gov/travel/destinationList.aspx for detail about vaccine and medicine prophylaxis recommendations.

Most Common Cause of Fever in Traveler (Central Asia)

Diagnosis or Illness[1]	% of all cases
No Cause Found	48%
Dengue	14%
Malaria	14%
Salmonella typhi or *Salmonella paratyphi*	14%
Mononucleosis (Epstein Barr or cytomegalovirus)	2%
Rickettsia	1%

Most Common Cause Acute Diarrhea in Traveler (Central Asia)

Diagnosis or Illness[1]	% of all cases
Parasite 　Giardia (29% of all diarrhea cases) 　Amoeba (10% of all diarrhea cases)	45%
Bacterial 　Campylobacter (9% of all diarrhea) 　Shigella (6% of all diarrhea) 　Non-typhoidal salmonella (1%a)	29%
Viral or No Cause Found	29%

Most Common Skin Disorders in Traveler (Central Asia)

Diagnosis or Illness[1]	% of all cases
Insect bite with/without infection	20%
Skin abscess or impetigo, erysipelas	19%
Allergic reaction or allergic rash	11%
Cutaneous Larva Migrans	6%
Mycosis (fungal)	6%
Mites (e.g. scabies)	3%
Leishmaniasis	2%
Swimmer's itch (Schistosomiasis)	< 1%
Myiasis	< 1%

Common Gastrointestinal Disorder–No Diarrhea (Central Asia)

Diagnosis or Illness[1]	% of all cases
Nematode/worms (Strongyloides, Ascaris)	31%
Gastritis or ulcer	9%
Hepatitis	8%

ASIA (SOUTHEAST/SE) TRAVELER

Most Common Cause of Fever in Traveler (SE Asia)

Diagnosis or Illness[1]	% of all cases
No Cause Found	45%
Dengue	32%
Malaria	13%
Mononucleosis (Epstein Barr or cytomegalovirus)	3%
Salmonella typhi or *Salmonella paratyphi*	3%
Rickettsia	2%

Most Common Cause of Acute Diarrhea in Traveler (SE Asia)

Diagnosis or Illness[1]	% of all cases
Viral or No Cause Found	40%

Bacterial
  Campylobacter (18% of all diarrhea)
  Non-typhoidal salmonella (6%)
  Shigella (3% of all diarrhea)
	37%

Parasite
  Giardia (12% of all diarrhea cases)
  Amoeba (7% of all diarrhea cases)
	26%

Most Common Skin Disorders in Traveler (SE Asia)

Diagnosis or Illness[1]	% of all cases
Insect bite with/without infection	18%
Cutaneous Larva Migrans	17%
Skin abscess or impetigo, erysipelas	14%
Allergic reaction or rash	9%
Mycosis (fungal)	6%
Mites (e.g. scabies)	2%
Swimmer's itch (Avian Schistosomiasis)	1%
Leishmaniasis	< 1%
Myiasis	< 1%

Most Common Gastrointestinal Disorder-No Diarrhea (SE Asia)

Diagnosis or Illness[1]	% of all cases
Nematode/worms (Strongyloides, Ascaris)	34%
Gastritis or ulcer	10%
Hepatitis	6%

AUSTRALIA & SOUTHWEST PACIFIC TRAVELER

Countries that Comprise the South West Pacific

American Samoa	Guam	Norfolk Island	Tahiti
	Kiribati	North Mariana	Tokelau
Australia	Marshall Isle(s)	Palau	Tonga
Christmas Isle	Micronesia	Papua	Tuvalu
Cocos Islands	Nauru	New Guinea	Vanuatu
Cook Islands	New Caledonia	Pitcairn Islands	Wake Island
Fiji	New Zealand	Samoa	Wallis &
Fr. Polynesia	Niue	Solomon Isle(s)	Futuna

Food/Waterborne Infections & Sanitation[1]

Clean water and sanitation are good in Australia and New Zealand and poor in other countries within this region.
Diarrhea due to parasites (esp. Entamoeba histolytic), bacteria, and viruses is common on less well developed islands.
Chronic *hepatitis* B occurs in > 8% on many Pacific islands while hepatitis C is present in up to 2% of all natives of this area.

Mosquito, Tick, & Flea borne Illness[1]

Malaria is found in Papua New Guinea, Vanuatu, and the Solomon islands. Dengue has been found throughout this region including northern Australia. Japanese encephalitis has been found in this region (esp. Papua New Guinea, Guam, western Pacific). Other diseases include scrub typhus, murine typhus, spotted fever, and Ross River fever.

Other Infectious Risks[1]

Other important diseases in this region include histoplasmosis, hookworm infections, leptospirosis, meliodosis, and strongyloidiasis.

---

[1] Disease lists are NOT all inclusive and leave out many common and unique diseases. See wwwn.cdc.gov/travel/destinationList.aspx for detail about vaccine and medicine prophylaxis recommendations.

CARIBBEAN TRAVELER

Countries that Comprise the Caribbean

Anguilla	Cuba	Martinique	St. Vincent &
Antigua	Dominica	Montserrat	Grenadines
& Barbuda	Dominican	Netherlands	Trinidad &
Aruba	Republic	Antilles	Tobago
Bahamas	Grenada	Puerto Rico	Turks & Caicos
Barbados	Guadeloupe	St Kitts & Nevis	Br Virgin Isl.
Bermuda	Haiti	St. Lucia	US Virgin
Caymans	Jamaica	St. Martin	Islands

Food/Waterborne Infections & Sanitation[1]

Clean water and sanitation levels vary between countries and water
and food-borne precautions should be maintained throughout most
travel. Certain high end resorts with their own water filtration and
cleansing systems usually can be relied upon to provide clean water.
Diarrhea due to bacteria (esp. Campylobacter, Salmonella, Shigella)
and parasites (esp., Giardia, Amoeba) is highest in the Dominican
Republic and Haiti although infectious diarrhea is prominent in many
Caribbean countries. *Hepatitis A* cases are particularly common in
the Dominican Republic and Haiti.

Mosquito, Tick, & Flea borne Illness[1]

Dengue fever is prominent in most of the Caribbean with recent
epidemics occurring in Cuba and Puerto Rico. *Leishmaniasis* is rare
except in Haiti and the Dominican Republic. Mosquitoes that carry
Malaria live in most islands of the Caribbean. Haiti and the
Dominican Republic have most cases while outbreaks and malaria
prophylaxis is recommended if traveling to these countries. Malaria
has occasionally occurred on other islands. *Yellow fever* has been
reported in the Caribbean and tick borne Rickettsia in Guadaloupe.

Other Infectious Risks[1]

Cutaneous larval migrans, leptospirosis, filariasis, HIV (2-7% risk in
Haiti) and ciguatera poisoning are other important disorders.

[1] Disease lists are NOT all inclusive and leave out many common
and unique diseases. See wwwn.cdc.gov/travel/destinationList.aspx
for detail about vaccine and medicine prophylaxis recommendations.

Most Common Cause of Fever (Caribbean Traveler)

Diagnosis or Illness[1]	% of all cases
No Cause Found	54%
Dengue	24%
Mononucleosis (Epstein Barr or cytomegalovirus)	7%
Malaria	7%
Salmonella typhi or *Salmonella paratyphi*	2%
Other diseases – each < 1% (e.g. Rickettsia)	< 1% each

Most Common Cause of Acute Diarrhea (Caribbean Traveler)

Diagnosis or Illness[1]	% of all cases
Viral illness or no cause found	48%

Parasite
  Giardia (13% of all diarrhea cases)
  Amoeba (11% of all diarrhea cases)
	28%

Bacterial
  Campylobacter (5% of all diarrhea)
  Shigella (4% of all diarrhea)
  Non-typhoidal salmonella (3% diarrhea)
	26%

Most Common Skin Disorders (Caribbean Traveler)

Diagnosis or Illness[1]	% of all cases
Cutaneous Larva Migrans	30%
Insect bite with/without associated infection	19%
Allergic reaction or allergic rash	15%
Skin abscess or impetigo, erysipelas	7%
Mycoses (fungal infection)	5%
Mites	3%
Swimmer's itch (Schistosomiasis)	< 1%
Leishmaniasis	0
Myiasis	0

Most Common Gastrointestinal Disorders Without Diarrhea

Diagnosis or Illness[1]	% of all cases
Nematode/worms (Strongyloides, Ascaris)	28%
Gastritis or ulcer	26%
Hepatitis	6%

CENTRAL AMERICA & MEXICO TRAVELER

Countries that Comprise Central America & Mexico

Belize	El Salvador	Honduras	Nicaragua
Costa Rica	Guatemala	Mexico	Panama

Food/Waterborne Infections & Sanitation[1]

Clean water and sanitation levels are poor and water and food-borne precautions should be maintained throughout most travel.

Diarrhea due to bacteria is most often caused by enterotoxigenic E. coli although many other bacteria and parasites are prevalent.

Hepatitis A is prevalent throughout Mexico and Central America. *Hepatitis E* epidemics have also occurred.

Mosquito, Tick, Fly, & Flea borne Illness[1]

Dengue is common throughout this region.

Mosquitoes that carry *malaria* live in Central America while Dengue fever is also common. Malaria is uncommon Mexico except on the West coast. As of early 2009, malaria chloroquine resistance was common in Panama while most other countries harbored chloroquine sensitive strains. Visitors to these areas require prophylaxis.

Yellow fever is especially prominent in Panama and travelers to some areas in this country require vaccination.

Other Infectious Risks[1]

Important diseases in this region include Chagas disease, cholera (esp. Nicaragua, Guatemala), coccidiomycosis, cysticercosis (a common cause of seizures in residents of this region), histoplasmosis, hookworms, leishmaniasis (sand fly), leptospirosis, murine typhus (flea), myiasis, onchocerciasis (black fly), rabies, relapsing fever (tick), and Strongyloidiasis.

[1] Disease lists are NOT all inclusive and leave out many common and unique diseases. See wwwn.cdc.gov/travel/destinationList.aspx for detail about vaccine and medicine prophylaxis recommendations.

Common Cause of Fever in Traveler (Mexico & Cent America)

Diagnosis or Illness[1]	% of all cases
No Cause Found	47%
Malaria	13%
Dengue	12%
Mononucleosis (Epstein Barr or cytomegalovirus)	7%
Salmonella typhi or *Salmonella paratyphi*	3%
Other diseases – each < 1% (e.g. Rickettsia)	< 1% each

Most Common Cause of Acute Diarrhea (Mexico-Cent America)

Diagnosis or Illness[1]	% of all cases
Viral illness or no cause found	40%
Parasite Amoeba (16% of all diarrhea cases) Giardia (14% of all diarrhea cases)	40%
Bacterial (Enterotoxigenic *E.coli* common) Campylobacter (3% of all diarrhea) Shigella (3% of all diarrhea) Non-typhoidal salmonella (1%)	19%

Common Skin Disorders in Traveler (Mexico & Cent America)

Diagnosis or Illness[1]	% of all cases
Insect bite with/without associated infection	24%
Cutaneous Larva Migrans	13%
Allergic reaction or allergic rash	13%
Myiasis	10%
Skin abscess or impetigo, erysipelas	7%
Leishmaniasis	6%
Mites (e.g. scabies)	4%
Mycosis (fungal)	3%
Swimmer's itch (Schistosomiasis)	0

Most Common Gastrointestinal Disorders Without Diarrhea

Diagnosis or Illness[1]	% of all cases
Nematodes/worms (Strongyloides, Ascaris)	27%
Gastritis or ulcer	9%
Hepatitis	9%

Countries that Comprise Western Europe

Andorra	France	Italy	Portugal
Austria	Germany	Liechtenstein	San Marino
Azores	Gibraltar	Luxembourg	Spain
Belgium	Greece	Malta	Sweden
Denmark	Greenland	Monaco	Switzerland
Faroe Islands	Iceland	Netherlands	United Kingdom
Finland	Ireland	Norway	Vatican

Food/Waterborne Infections & Sanitation[1]

Clean water and sanitation are uniformly present although rare outbreaks of diarrhea can occur. Brucellosis occurs in countries that abut the Mediterranean from handling animals or via unpasteurized milk or milk products.

Hepatitis A is prevalent in Greenland.

Mosquito, Tick, Fly, & Flea borne Illness[1]

Mosquitoes borne illness is rare in Europe. Tick borne diseases including *Lyme* and *tick born encephalitis* are present. Leishmaniasis is prominent in countries abutting the Mediterranean.

Other Infectious Risks[1]

Important diseases in this region include echinococcus (Mediterranean countries), Q fever (Mediterranean), rabies, and tularemia (esp. Sweden, France, Spain).

[1] Disease lists are NOT all inclusive and leave out many common and unique diseases. See wwwn.cdc.gov/travel/destinationList.aspx for detail about vaccine and medicine prophylaxis recommendations.

Countries that Comprise Eastern Europe & Northern Asia

Albania	Czech	Lithuania	Slovakia
Armenia	Republic	Macedonia	Slovenia
Azerbaijan	Estonia	Moldova	Tajikistan
Belarus	Georgia	Montenegro	Turkmenistan
Bosnia &	Hungary	Poland	Ukraine
Herzegovina	Kazakhstan	Romania	Uzbekistan
Bulgaria	Kyrgyzstan	Russia	
Croatia	Latvia	Serbia	

Food/Waterborne Infections & Sanitation[1]

Clean water and sanitation are usually poor in these countries.

Hepatitis A is prevalent in many countries in this region. Hepatitis E is also a risk in southern Russia.

Mosquito, Tick, Fly, & Flea borne Illness[1]

Malaria occurs in the south of this region (Armenia, Azerbaijan, Georgia, Tajikistan, Turkmenistan, Uzbekistan) during warmer months.

Tick borne encephalitis occurs in the forested regions of Europe and Asia that do not lie within the tropics (esp. Czech Republic, Estonia, Hungary, Latvia, Lithuania, Poland, Russia, Slovenia). Lyme disease (former Soviet Union), murine typhus (flea), scrub typhus (chigger), spotted fever (tick), and relapsing fever (tick) occur in parts of this region. Japanese encephalitis (mosquito) is found in eastern Russia.

Other Infectious Risks[1]

Important diseases occurring in this region include botulism, brucellosis, Q fever, rabies, tuberculosis (drug resistant), and typhoid fever.

[1] Disease lists are NOT all inclusive and leave out many common and unique diseases. See wwwn.cdc.gov/travel/destinationList.aspx for detail about vaccine and medicine prophylaxis recommendations.

Countries that Comprise the Middle East

Bahrain	Israel	Oman	Turkey
Cyprus	Jordan	Qatar	United Arab
Iran	Kuwait	Saudi Arabia	Emirates
Iraq	Lebanon	Syria	Yemen

Food/Waterborne Infections & Sanitation[1]

Clean water and sanitation are sporadic with most water in Bahrain, Cyprus, and Israel safe to drink.

Diarrhea due to bacteria, parasites, and viruses is prominent. In 2004, outbreaks of cholera were reported in Iran and Iraq.

Hepatitis A and *B* are prevalent in this region and vaccination against both viruses is recommended prior to travel.

Mosquito, Tick, Fly, & Flea borne Illness[1]

Malaria is sporadically present in areas of Iran, Iraq, Oman, Saudi Arabia (southern), Syria, Turkey, and Yemen and prophylaxis is recommended if traveling to malaria endemic regions within these countries. Chloroquine resistance is reported in Iran, Saudi Arabia, and Yemen).

Dengue epidemics have occurred in Saudi Arabia, and Yemen.

Leishmaniasis (sand fly) is widespread, especially in areas that lie on the Mediterranean sea.

Other infections include filariasis (mosquito), murine typhus (flea), onchocerciasis (black fly), relapsing fever (tick), spotted fever (tick).

Other Infectious Risks[1]

Important diseases occurring in this region include anthrax (esp. Turkey), brucellosis, echinococcosis, polio, meningitis due to *Neisseria meningitidis* (esp. pilgrims to the Hajj in Saudi Arabia), plague, Q fever, rabies, tuberculosis, and worms (hookworms, tapeworms).

[1] Disease lists are NOT all inclusive and leave out many common and unique diseases. See wwwn.cdc.gov/travel/destinationList.aspx for detail about vaccine and medicine prophylaxis recommendations.

SOUTH AMERICA TRAVELER

Countries that Comprise South America

Argentina	Easter Island	Galapagos	South Sandwich
Bolivia	Ecuador	Guyana	Islands
Brazil	Falkland	Paraguay	Suriname
Chile	Islands	Peru	Uruguay
Colombia	French Guiana	South Georgia	Venezuela

Tropical S. America - (all areas north of Argentina, Chile, Uruguay)

Food/Waterborne Infections & Sanitation[1]

Clean water and sanitation is sporadic in South America. Cholera used to be widespread and only recently has been limited to Brazil, Colombia, and Ecuador. Typhoid fever has occurred sporadically throughout S. American and has been epidemic in Chile and Peru. *Hepatitis A and B* are common in South America. Vaccination against both viruses is recommended.

Mosquito, Tick, & Flea borne Illness[1]

Malaria occurs in most tropical countries in South America (esp. Brazil, Bolivia, Colombia, Ecuador, French Guiana, Guiana, Peru, and Venezuela). Prophylaxis (see pages 99-101) is recommended for these areas. Chloroquine resistance medicines are especially required in the Amazon Basin and increasingly in other regions. *Dengue fever* is prevalent throughout most of South America. *Yellow fever* is present in most tropical areas of South America (north of Argentina, Chile, Uruguay). Vaccination is recommended if travel to rural or jungle areas in tropical South America.

Other Infectious Risks[1]

Important diseases occurring in this region include Bartonellosis (Oroya fever) in the Andes, Chagas disease, Filariasis, Leishmaniasis (tropical South America), Onchocerciasis, Schistosomiasis

[1] Disease lists are NOT all inclusive and leave out many common and unique diseases. See www.cdc.gov/travel/destinationList.aspx for detail about vaccine and medicine prophylaxis recommendations.

Most Common Cause of Fever in Traveler

Diagnosis or Illness[1]	% of all cases
No Cause Found	55%
Dengue	14%
Malaria	13%
Mononucleosis (Epstein Barr or cytomegalovirus)	8%
Salmonella typhi or *Salmonella paratyphi*	2%
Other diseases – each < 1% (e.g. Rickettsia)	< 1% each

Most Common Cause of Acute Diarrhea in Traveler

Diagnosis or Illness[1]	% of all cases
Viral illness or no cause found	38%

Parasite
    Giardia (16% of all diarrhea cases)
    Amoeba (14% of all diarrhea cases)
	37%

Bacterial (Enterotoxigenic *E.coli* common)
    Campylobacter (9% of all diarrhea)
    Shigella (4% of all diarrhea)
    Non-typhoidal salmonella (1%)
	25%

Most Common Skin Disorders in Traveler

Diagnosis or Illness[1]	% of all cases
Insect bite with/without associated infection	16%
Leishmaniasis	14%
Cutaneous Larva Migrans	12%
Allergic reaction or allergic rash	10%
Myiasis	10%
Skin abscess or impetigo, erysipelas	6%
Mites (e.g. scabies)	4%
Mycosis (fungal)	4%
Swimmer's itch (Schistosomiasis)	< 1%

Most Common Gastrointestinal Disorders Without Diarrhea

Diagnosis or Illness[1]	% of all cases
Nematodes/worms (Strongyloides, Ascaris)	26%
Gastritis or ulcer	17%
Hepatitis	10%

Allergy & Anaphylaxis

Background:

- The most common causes of severe allergy are penicillin, aspirin, bee/wasp stings, nuts, shellfish, milk, eggs and latex.
- People with asthma, asthma in their family, or atopic dermatitis (eczema) have an increased risk of developing allergic reactions.

Features: Symptoms of allergic reactions can be mild and confined to a local rash (hives) with red raised areas, runny nose, or itchy eyes or can be severe or life-threatening (anaphylaxis). Severe symptoms include throat closure, wheezing, shortness of breath, light headedness or black out due to a drop in blood pressure, or a change in mental status. Other severe symptoms that are less well recognized as allergic include abdomen pain, vomiting, diarrhea, and chest pain.

Prevention & Treatment: Seek medical care in all but mild cases

Skin Reactions (*see page 55 for insect sting care*)	• Oral histamine 1 (H1) blocker - diphenhydramine (*Benadryl*) – 25 to 50 mg or 1 mg/kg orally for children (max. dose 50 mg) used every 4-6 hours • Oral H2 blocker - cimetidine (*Tagamet*) 300 mg or famotidine (*Pepcid*) 20 mg twice/day • Oral steroids (prednisone 1 mg/kg) daily
Wheezing[1]	• Albuterol nebulizer or inhalant every 4 hours • Epinephrine (1:1000) – 0.01 mg/kg intramuscular (maximum 0.4 mg) if no inhalants are available • Steroids oral or via intravenous line • H2 blockers may worsen wheezing
Anaphylaxis[1]	• Lie patient down to treat falling/lightheadedness • Epinephrine (1:1000) – 0.01 mg/kg intramuscular IM deltoid or lateral thigh (maximum 0.4 mg) • Intravenous (IV) fluids for low blood pressure • IV diphenhydramine (*Benadryl*) • Intravenous or oral steroids

[1]Epinephrine can increase blood pressure and worsen heart disease. *EpiPen* is an autoinjector that delivers 0.3 mg epinephrine IM *EpiPen Jr.* is an autoinjector that delivers 0.15 mg epinephrine IM for children weighing 33 to 66 pounds (15 and 30 kilograms)

HIGH ALTITUDE ILLNESS

High altitude is defined as 1500 to 3500 meters (~5000-10,000 feet) above sea level; Very high altitude is 3500 to 5500 meters (~10,000-18,000 feet) above sea level; and Extreme altitude is a height > 5500 meters (> 18,000 feet) above sea level. High altitude causes a drop in the blood's oxygen saturation to less than 90% (normal is > 95%) in individuals who are above 8,000 to 10,000 feet or at lower altitudes in those with underlying heart, lung, or blood disorders. High altitude can cause minor or life threatening disorders including acute mountain sickness (AMS), retinopathy (bleeding in back of eye), high altitude pulmonary edema (HAPE) or fluid in the lungs, and high altitude cerebral edema (HACE) or swelling in the brain. To avoid these disorders, travelers must be aware of the altitudes to which they are traveling, preventative measures, how to identify onset of disease, and what to do if a high altitude syndrome develops.

Prevention of Altitude Illness

Do not ascend quickly to sleeping altitude > 3000 meters (10,000 ft) & Do not increase sleeping altitude > 500 meters/day above 3000 meters
Spend 72 hours at 2500 meters (8200 feet) before going higher
Mild exercise may aid in acclimatization (do not overexert)
Drink plenty of fluids & eat foods that are high in carbohydrates
Do not use sedatives, alcohol, cigarettes, or sleep aids
Consider prophylactic medicines[1] with your doctor

[1] See table page 50, for medication options

Acute Mountain Sickness (AMS)

AMS occurs soon after rapidly ascending with up to ¼ developing at an altitude > 2500 meters (> 8200 feet).

Features: Headache is universally present. It is throbbing, worse at night, with arising in the morning, or with abruptly sitting/standing. Other symptoms include nausea, vomiting, weakness, fatigue, dizziness, and trouble sleeping.

Management: Mild cases require stopping the ascent or descent to a lower altitude for sleeping. Other treatments include nausea medications, acetazolamide (*Diamox*), oxygen, and dexamethasone for more severe cases. (See table, page 50) Close observation and acute intervention are required if high altitude pulmonary edema or high altitude cerebral edema are suspected. See pages 49 and 50.

High Altitude Pulmonary Edema (HAPE)

HAPE is the most common cause of death due to high altitude illness. This disorder is due to leak of fluid from the capillaries into the airspaces of the lungs. It is rare below 2500 meters (8200 feet) with uncommon cases between 2500-3000 meters due to heavy exercise. HAPE primarily occurs at altitudes > 4200 meters (> 14,000 feet). Unlike AMS, HAPE can take 2-4 days to develop.

Features: HAPE causes a cough with clear or pink/bloody sputum, shortness of breath, a rapid respiratory rate, and rapid heart rate. Shortness of breath that occurs while at rest should ALWAYS be considered a sign of impending HAPE. Cyanosis (blue nail-beds or lips) may be present. Symptoms of AMS often coexist (e.g. headache, weakness, fatigue, nausea).

Management: Immediate descent to a lower altitude, avoiding exercise, and oxygen (hyperbaric or pressurized) are required if HAPE is suspected. Hospitalization and use of a variety of medications are standard. (Table, page 50)

High Altitude Cerebral Edema (HACE)

HACE (or swelling of the brain) primarily occurs at elevations above 3500 meters (11,500 feet). Onset of symptoms to development of coma can take from 12 hours to 1 week. AMS & HAPE can coexist.

Features: Symptoms include incoordination (early), slurred speech, an altered mental status, stroke like symptoms, and eventual coma.

Management: Treatment includes rapid descent, oxygen, and dexamethasone (*Decadron*) therapy (Table, page 50) After descent, intensive care admission with other measures to decrease intracranial pressure (furosemide, mannitol) is required.

Other Disorders: All travelers who ascend to high altitudes should be aware that low oxygen and low pressures can worsen underlying, hypertension, cardiovascular disease, and lung disease. Travelers with sickle cell trait may experience vaso-occlusive crises and infarction of the spleen especially with exertion. At extreme elevations, bleeding within the retina (the posterior part of the eye) may occur. Fortunately, visual loss does not always occur and symptoms may resolve within a few weeks. Travelers with prior corneal surgery may experience uneven swelling of the cornea at high altitudes with resulting visual blurring.

Treatment Options - High Altitude Illness

Intervention	Use in[1]	Specifics
Descent	ALL	Descent of as little as 500-1000 meters may be life saving
Rest & Warmth	ALL	Exercise and Hypothermia can worsen high altitude illness
Oxygen	ALL	
Hyperbaric Oxygen (Not a substitute for descent)	HACE HAPE	Portable chambers/bags are available that can pressurize to an equivalent of descending 1500-2500 meters. Inflate to 2 psi (104 mm Hg) and treat for 1 hour at time while continually pumping to prevent CO_2 buildup.
Medications (Adult Dosing – Discuss with your doctor)[2,3,4]		
Acetazolamide (*Diamox*)	ALL	*Prevention* 125-125 mg PO twice/day Treatment -250 mg PO twice per day
Dexamethasone (*Decadron*)	Severe AMS HACE	AMS: 4 mg PO every 6 hours HACE: 8 mg PO, then 4 mg PO every 6 hours
Furosemide (*Lasix*)	HAPE	Given at 0.5 to 1 mg per kilogram IV when hospitalized
Mannitol		Given IV when hospitalized
Nifedipine (*Procardia*)	HAPE	Treatment & Prevention: 20 to 30 mg of sustained release pill every 12 hours
Salmeterol (*Serevent*)	HAPE	*Prevention* - 125 mcg inhaled every 12 hours
Sildenafil (*Viagra*)	HAPE	*Prevention* – 50 mg PO every 8 hours Treatment dose unknown
Tadalafil (*Cialis*)	HAPE	*Prevention* – 10 mg PO every 12 hours Treatment dose unknown

[1] ALL – AMS (acute mountain sickness), HACE (high altitude cerebral edema), and HAPE (high altitude pulmonary edema)
[2] Multiple serious side effects and drug interactions. Discuss use of these medications with medical experts BEFORE traveling to high altitudes and BEFORE use at high altitudes when possible.
[3] Treatment dose unless specified as *prevention*. Prevention dosing begins 1-2 days pre-ascent and is continued 2 days post ascent.
[4] mg – milligrams, mcg – micrograms, PO orally, IV - intravenous

BITES & STINGS
Animal bites & Rabies

Background:

- Wild animals rarely attack humans unless they are provoked, they have rabies, or they are large carnivores (meat eaters).
- Suturing any animal bite can increase the risk of infection.
- While rabies is most common in tropical and subtropical regions of the world, it occurs in all continents except Antarctica.
- Rabies has been isolated from all mammals (and many bats), is most common in carnivores and is rare in rodents & rabbits.

Features: The most important concerns with animal bites are direct trauma, infections, and disease transmission (i.e. rabies, plague, murine typhus, rat bite fever).

Infection: Localized infection occurs in up to half of all cat bites and scratches, 1/3 of dog bites, and as few as 2% of rodent bites. The infection risk is increased if the hand, wrist, foot, or a joint is involved. Punctures and crush injuries are more likely to cause infection than scrapes and simple lacerations. Infection risk is increased for victims older than 50 years, or who have diabetes, vascular disease, or who have a weakened immune system.

Rabies: Rabies is disease affecting the brain caused by a virus that is transmitted by the saliva of a large variety of animals across all continents except Antarctica. In the United States, Hawaii is the only state that had no reported animals or bats with rabies as of 2008. Rabies infection has an incubation period of 1-3 months. Patients 1st develop fever, headache, sore throat, & muscle pain. Then, spasm of swallowing muscles, weakness, paralysis, and mental status changes develop. Eventually coma & death occur in almost all cases.

While all mammals can contract and transmit rabies, bats and dogs are the most important carriers of this disease. In the United States, Asia, Africa, and Latin America, dogs are a common carrier. In Europe, Canada, and the Arctic/sub-Arctic regions, the fox is the most common carrier. Other common and important reservoirs are raccoons, coyotes, skunks, foxes, bats, jackals, and the mongoose. Any scratch, bite, or exposure to animal saliva can transmit rabies. Cases of possible airborne rabies are described in adults who were in caves or who slept in a room where a bat resided even though no documented bite occurred.

Other Infections Transmitted by Animals: Multiple exotic infections can be transmitted by contact with the skin or body fluids or animals or by the fleas that they carry (see pages 56-61). Specific infections include Brucellosis (deer, fox, raccoons), Leptospirosis (skunks, foxes, raccoons, rodents), Salmonella (birds, reptiles), Tularemia (rabbits), Tetanus (ubiquitous in the environment), Psittacosis (birds), Rat bite fever. Multiple symptoms occur depending upon the infecting organisms and degree of infection including but not limited to fever, respiratory or gastrointestinal symptoms, rash, muscle or joint pain.

Treatment: Major trauma victims require basic life support (page 119) and rapid transport to a medical facility. Minor trauma requires and evaluation of the injury and assessment of risk for local infection and disease transmission.

Wound care: All wounds require evaluation for trauma to underlying structures including tendons, bone, joint and blood vessel injury and exclusion of retained foreign bodies. X-rays may be required to exclude foreign bodies or underlying fractures. While significant wounds generally require evaluation at a medical facility, early cleansing and irrigation can greatly decrease the chance of a localized infection and can reduce the chance of acquiring rabies and other viruses. Rinsing or irrigation with soap & water, a povidone-iodine solution, or 1-2% benzalkonium chloride solution will kill most bacteria and viruses including rabies. Importantly, closing or suturing a wound does not decrease and in many instances will increase the probability that an infection will occur.

Antibiotics are advised for high risk wounds. Recommended oral antibiotics for most bites include amoxicillin with clavulanate (*Augmentin*) or doxycycline. Alternatives include cefuroxime (*Ceftin*) for cat bites, and clindamycin (*Cleocin*) plus ciprofloxacin (*Cipro*) for dog bites. Methicillin resistant *Staphylococcus aureus* (MRSA) is becoming common after skin trauma and can be treated with trimethoprim-sulfamethoxazole (*Bactrim* or *Septra*), clindamycin, or linezolid. Intravenous antibiotics may be required for moderate to severe infections, heavily traumatized wounds, or victims with underlying vascular disease or who are immunocompromised.

Tetanus Prevention: Tetanus is a disease manifesting as muscle spasms and seizure like activity due to bacteria that live in most soil and almost everywhere within the environment. While localized cleansing of wounds can diminish the probability of developing tetanus, vaccination is the most important preventative measure travelers can undergo to prevent this disease. Importantly, if travelers have had 3 or more tetanus vaccines with the latest within the past 5 years, they will require no tetanus vaccine or immune globulin if a wound occurs during travel.

Tetanus Immunization Recommendations

Victim Immune Status	*Tetanus prone Wounds*	*Non-tetanus prone Wounds (Clean & Minor)*
Victim has had < 3 prior vaccinations	Td[1] TIG[2]	Td[1]
Victim has had 3 or more prior tetanus vaccinations	Td[1] if > 5 years since last dose	Td[1] if > 10 years since last dose

[1] Vaccine types include Td, DT, DTaP, and Tdap. Use Tdap (*Adacel*) for 1st dose if no prior Tdap & 7 to 64 years old. Td is preferred in pregnancy although Tdap is not contraindicated. If given, administration in 2nd, 3rd trimester is preferred. If < 7 years old, use DT (different dose of D-diphtheria component) or DTaP (DT with aP – acellular pertussis component).

[2] Tetanus immune globulin. Dose – 250 units intramuscular (IM) at site other than for Td/Tdap OR if < 7 years old, use 4 units/kg IM.

Rabies prevention, Pre-exposure: For travelers who spend a prolonged amount of time in locations (e.g. wildlife workers, sperlunkers) with a high rabies risk and where medical resources are limited, vaccination prior to travel is advised. For these individuals, a vaccine used in the US (HDCV – human diploid cell vaccine or PCEC – purified chick embryo cell vaccine) is given on days 0, 7, and 21 or 28. If a rabies exposure occurs, a booster vaccine is required at day 0 and day 3 after exposure but immune globulin is not required.

Rabies prevention, Post-exposure

WHO Rabies Exposure Categories	• Category I – Touch, feeding, licking intact skin • Category II – Nibbling uncovered skin, minor scratches or abrasions without bleeding, licks on broken skin • Category III – bite/bites or contamination of scratches or mucous membranes with saliva
Wound care	• Immediate washing/scrubbing of the wound with soap & water. If puncture, swab deep at edges. • Next, scrub with benzalkonium chloride (1-2%) or povidone-iodine (or ethanol 700 ml/Liter)
Animal observation	• In US, if cat, dog, or ferret can be captured, it is observed for 10 days. If the animal dies or develops symptoms, it is sacrificed and tested. • In other countries, the World Health Organization (WHO) recommends deferring treatment while observing the animal ONLY if (1) rabies is uncommon in the species and the lab diagnosis can be made within 48 hours of the bite, or (2) if the exposure involved a dog > 1 year old with a current vaccination that can be observed for 10 days. If the dog develops symptoms, treatment is begun rather than waiting for test results.
Rabies Immune globulin (RIG)	• Human RIG intramuscularly/IM into/around wound (20 Units/kg) Or equine RIG 40 units/kg • If unable to give all at wound site, administer remainder at a site distant from wound • WHO only recommends RIG for Category III exposures due to limited RIG availability
Vaccine[1]	• Classic (Essen) regimen – 1 milliliter of vaccine is given in deltoid muscle or lateral thigh in children (NOT buttocks) on days 0, 3, 7 and 14

[1] When vaccine availability is limited, WHO recommends intradermal (ID) regimen of human diploid cell (HDCV) or purified chick embryo vaccine (PCECV) 0.1 ml each at 8 sites (arms, legs, abdomen, supra-scapular) on day 0, **4 shots (4 sites)** on day 7, & 1 shot on day 28 & 90. **OR** 2 intradermal shots (HDCV, PCECV, or purified vero cell vaccine) are given on days 0, 3, 7 & 1 shot is given on day 28 and 90.

Ants, Bees, Hornets, and Wasps

Background:
- Ants, bees, and wasps can deliver venom by biting, stinging, or secretions through pores or hairs.
- Deaths from stinging insects are more common than from snake bites in developed countries.

Features: These insects can cause local irritation or an allergic reaction that is localized or diffuse (anaphylaxis). Skin effects include hives (urticaria), itching, pain, redness, and swelling of the affected site. Serious symptoms (See anaphylaxis, page 47) include throat tightness or closure, wheezing, breathing difficulty, abdomen pain, vomiting, chest pain, lightheadedness or blacking out.

Treatment & Prevention: Most bees, hornets, and wasps sting to protect their colony, or hive. Loud activity, bright or dark colors and certain smells (e.g. perfume) attract these insects and may lead to stings. When threatened, these insects release hormones that attract other colony members and incite them to sting.

Insect Sting or Bite Treatment

Wound Care	• Apply ice • Remove stinger by gentle scraping with flat object that is parallel to skin or by pinching or grasping and pulling. • Remove stinger as rapidly as possible as venom is injected for up to one minute after sting • Clean area with soap and water
Medications (See page 47)	• Oral antihistamines for local or skin reactions • Oral steroids (prednisone) for minor reactions • Inhaled β_2 agonists (albuterol) for wheezing • Epinephrine IM for severe reactions • Intravenous fluids for low blood pressure
Delayed symptoms	• Continue antihistamines and steroids for 3 days after sting to prevent relapse of symptoms • Redness and warmth that begins > 24 hours after the sting or that begins early and persists > 72 hours may signify a skin infection (cellulitis) • Delayed serum sickness (joint and muscle pain) can develop up to 2 weeks after the 1st sting

Bed bugs
Background:
- Beg bugs are most common in tropical and subtropical regions.
- Bed bugs are 3 to 6 mm in length and cannot fly or jump.
- Bed bugs feed at night and live within clothes, bedding, and luggage.

Features: Bed bug bites are usually painless. Symptoms occur after the bite due to local irritation and a localized allergic reaction or hives. A secondary skin infection may develop days after the bite if the skin is traumatized from scratching or if large blisters occur.

Treatment: No specific treatment is needed for the bites. Oral or topical antihistamines (diphenhydramine/*Benadryl*, cetirizine/*Zyrtec*, loratadine/*Claritin*) and topical steroids may relieve itching.

Bugs, Fleas, & Flies
Background:
- Fleas can transmit plaque (bubonic plague) and murine typhus from rats to humans.
- Disease transmission from fleas can either be from a flea bite, or rat feces carried by fleas that is either inhaled or that comes into contact with unintact skin.
- Sand fleas, also known as jigger or chigoe, cause an infestation and infection of the foot known as tungiasis in those who walk barefoot in endemic areas.
- Tsetse flies causing African trypanosomiasis (sleeping sickness) are attracted to bright colors. For this reason, thick olive or khaki clothes are recommended when traveling to endemic areas.
- Treatment for many diseases transmitted by bites of arthropods (bugs, flies, fleas) can be complex and will usually require management by travel medicine or infectious disease experts.

Features:

Bubonic plague is caused by a bacteria (*Yersinia pestis*) that is transmitted by the bite of infected fleas that are carried by rodents. The pneumonic (lung infection) form can be passed between humans via inhalation of infected droplets. Natural plague is found in semi-arid areas of Asia, Eastern Europe, Africa, South and North America. Outbreaks occur mostly in rural locations where infected rodents are found. Symptoms begin within 2-6 days of exposure. Large painful lymph nodes near the point of entry (buboes in bubonic plague), pneumonia (pneumonic plague), and disseminated blood stream infections (septicemic plague) can occur. Bubonic plague results in fever, chills, headache, muscle aches, bleeding from any site, cough, respiratory difficulty and eventual shock. Darkened skin lesions from bleeding under the skin were responsible for the plague being known as Black Death during the Middle Ages.

Chagas disease, also known as American trypanosomiasis, is caused by the parasite *Trypanosoma cruzi* which is transmitted by the feces of reduviid (or triatomine) bugs. Rare cases occur after blood transfusion and organ transplantation. Chagas disease is found throughout Mexico, Central, and South America. The reduviid bug lives in mud & adobe walls and thatched or bamboo roofs and is especially common in poor and rural areas. This insect often will bite the face, arm, or another site of a victim at night leaving behind the parasite in its feces. Scratching or rubbing the area will introduce the parasite into the blood stream. After a bite, travelers may develop a red nodule with swelling around at the site. A common scenario is swelling around the eye, eye injection/irritation (conjunctivitis), and lymph nodes in front of the ear. Within days, fever, weakness, lymph nodes throughout the body, myocarditis (inflamed heart muscle with difficulty breathing, chest pain), or encephalitis/meningitis (inflammation of brain tissue or its surround layer with headache, altered mentation, vomiting, neck stiffness) may develop. In many cases, acute symptoms resolve within 1-3 months. In ¼ of all cases, cardiomyopathy (a weakened heart muscle with heart failure or fluid build-up in lungs), or massive dilation of the esophagus or colon (vomiting, abdominal pain, and other digestive symptoms) develops years after the initial infection.

Myiasis is a disorder causes by fly larvae burrowing on or near open wounds producing open wounds. Wounds that look like boils appear at the site of burrowing. These wounds may have a sensation of movement with pain but little inflammation. The tip of the larva may be seen at the central opening accompanied by occasional bubbles. Wounds can be confused with leishmaniasis and onchocerciasis which must be excluded.

Onchocerciasis is a parasitic disease caused by a nematode. This parasite is transmitted by black flies which breed in well oxygenated water found in rivers and streams. The disease is found in 38 countries within Africa (esp. Western and sub-Saharan), South America, and the Middle East. While this disease can affect any organ, skin findings and blindness (river blindness) are most common. The initial bite of the black fly often goes unnoticed. Within 1-2 years, larvae migrate and develop into adult worms. Itching can be severe and lead to chronic ulcers and resulting skin infections. In West Africa, this is called "craw-craw". Skin loses its pigment over time and can become pale especially in the shins causing "leopard skin". Swollen lymph nodes are often found near the sites of infection. Visual symptoms include redness, itching, blurring, sensitivity to light, and eventual visual loss. The cornea eventually becomes cloudy with eventual glaucoma (increased pressure) and cataract development.

Sand flies: Female sand flies feed on blood, mostly during calm, windless nights with most bites occurring on the face or neck. Two important diseases transmitted by sand flies include leishmaniasis and bartonellosis (diseases from Bartonella bacteria). **Leishmaniasis** is a disease that occurs from parasites transmitted via sand fly bites that occurs primarily in Central America, South America, the Middle East, Africa, India, Asia, southern Europe and the Mediterranean. Symptoms can manifest with skin lesions (cutaneous leishmaniasis), mucous membrane lesions (mucocutaneous leishmaniasis) or the disease can involve internal organs (visceral leishmaniasis). Cutaneous leishmaniasis is most common in Afghanistan, Brazil, Iran, Iraq, Peru, and Saudi Arabia while visceral disease is most common in Bangladesh, Brazil, India, Nepal, and the Sudan.

Skin lesions are initially red raised areas < 2-3 centimeters in diameter. Eventual crusting, then ulceration occurs with eventual healing of the ulcers and scarring within 3-6 months. Mucous membranes (e.g. lips, palate, nose) can ulcerate and become eroded. With visceral disease, fever, weight loss, diarrhea, general darkening of the skin, and liver and spleen enlargement occur. Secondary bacterial infections, tuberculosis, dysentery, anemia, and bleeding can occur with eventual death.

Bartonellosis - While there are multiple diseases caused by Bartonella species, the sand fly transmits the species that causes Oroya fever (also called Carrion disease). Oroya fever is primarily limited to South American, especially within the Andes mountains. Illness often begins with a fever 3-12 weeks after a sand fly bite. Chills, headache, sweating, mental status changes and seizures can occur. In 1/3 of cases, a secondary infection by Salmonella species or other organisms occurs. Skin eruptions (verruga peruana) also can occur weeks to months after the initial illness with small vascular nodules that grow, ulcerate, bleed, and scar.

Tsetse flies carry the parasite (*Trypanosoma brucei*) which is responsible for African trypanosomiasis or sleeping sickness. Symptoms occur after the parasite is transmitted via the bite of infected tsetse flies which are only found only in Africa. This disease is confined primarily to tropical Africa between latitudes 15°N and 20°S or from the northern part of South Africa to just south of Algeria, Libya, and Egypt. The tsetse fly rests in bushes and will bite if disturbed. It is also attracted to bright and very dark colors and dust that moving vehicles and animals cause. It can bite through thin fabrics. Early symptoms include a painless sore beginning 5-15 days after the bite at the site of the tsetse fly bite. There is an early fever, muscle aches, and headache 2-3 weeks after the bite. Lymph nodes throughout the body become swollen. Groin and axillary (armpit) lymph nodes are more common in the Eastern African form while cervical (neck) nodes are more common with the Western African form. Later (months to a year later), symptoms of central nervous system (brain) involvement occur with headaches, irritability, tremors, increased muscle tone and rigidity, daytime sleepiness, nighttime insomnia, depression, mood swings, psychosis, weight loss, seizures, and coma.

Tungiasis is an infestation by human fleas also known as sand fleas, chigger fleas, jigger, nigua, pigue, and le bicho de pe. These fleas often burrow into the skin on the bottom of the foot causing ulcers, nodules, scarring and secondary skin infections. Other body sites coming in contact with the beach can become infected. Tiny black spots can be seen at the site of the skin penetration. Tungiasis is common in Central America, the Caribbean, South America, India, and tropical Africa.

Prevention & Treatment: For each of these infestations and infection, the most important step is to avoid areas & environments with high risk for bite from the fleas, flies, or bugs that carry infection. Appropriate netting, clothing (thick, tan or khaki and no bright colors), insect repellant, and insecticides will also decrease the risk of acquiring many of these infections. (See malaria prevention, page 99-101)

Bubonic plague – An inactivated vaccine is available for <u>preventing</u> disease in high risk populations (esp. laboratory or field personnel who will be exposed to rodents with *Yersinia pestis*). However, the vaccine is not completely effective, severe reactions can occur, and boosters are required at frequent intervals. Travelers with <u>exposure</u> but no disease can be treated with 7 days of oral doxycycline or ciprofloxacin. <u>Disease</u> is treated with 10 days of streptomycin given as an intramuscular injection or with 10 days of intravenous gentamicin, ciprofloxacin, or doxycycline.

Chagas disease – Treatment of the acute phase consists of nifurtimox (*Lampit*) which is only available in the US from the Centers for Disease Control or benznidazole (*Rochagan, Radanil*) available outside of the US. Infectious disease, tropical medicine, or travel medicine experts should direct the care of travelers when Chagas disease is suspected. Congenital disease (mother to baby) and recurrent or chronic disease in immunocompromised patients also require treatment with these agents.

Myiasis can be treated in a variety of manners. One unproven remedy involved binding a piece of fat or bacon over the opening of the wound causing the larva to leave their burrow. Alternately, a local anesthetic can be injected into the base of the wound causing pressure that extrudes the larva. Surgical excision also may be required.

Onchocerciasis is treated with ivermectin (*Stromectol*) 150 micrograms per kilogram administered every 3-12 months. This agent does not kill adult parasites but stops disease progression. Doxycycline suppresses disease progression but has not been proven superior to ivermectin. Another agent, suramin (*Germanin*), may kill adult parasites but significant toxicity limits its use.

Sand flies –Treatment of cutaneous leishmaniasis includes topical paromomycin for mild disease while more severe disease requires sodium stibogluconate, meglumine antimonite, or pentamidine. Mucousal disease requires pentavalent antimony or amphotericin B. Visceral leishmaniasis management requires treatment of underlying complications (e.g. bacterial infection, anemia) and antimicrobials including pentavelent antimony, amphotericin B, or miltefosine (*Impavido, Miltex*) which is primarily available in South America, India, and Germany.
Treatment of Oroya fever consists of doxycycline, ciprofloxacin, ampicillin, or trimethoprim-sulfamethoxazole. Rifampin can be used for isolated skin disease (verruga peruana).

Tsetse flies. No vaccine or medication is currently recommended to prevent disease. Several agents are effective in treating sleeping sickness including suramin, pentamidine, melarsoprol, eflornithine, and nifurtimox depending upon the strain of organism, and the state of disease. Treatment regimens are relatively toxic and underlying nutritional deficiencies and potential coexisting infections also may require treatment (e.g. helminths/worms, malaria)

Tungiasis can be prevented by wearing shoes on beaches and not sitting or lying on the beach. Thiabendazole or ivermectin lotion applied on 2 consecutive days can eradicate this disease. Secondary bacterial infections may require antibiotics.

Mites - Scabies

Background:
- Human scabies is a highly contagious infestation due to mites.
- Most cases are due to personal contact with infected persons.
- Mites can live on objects for up to one week. They do NOT jump.

Features: Infestations cause an intense itching that is worse at night. Skin lesions occur on the hands' web spaces (between the fingers), the wrist, elbows, armpit, groin & buttocks. Small red raised 1-3 millimeter areas form a small burrowing trail under the skin. Crusted scabies, also known as Norwegian scabies, causes skin thickening, crusting, and scaling with less intense itching. Crusted scabies are more common in immunocompromised individuals and can lead to infestations with up to one million mites. Secondary skin infections (page 113) can occur due to skin breakdown and repeated scratching.

Prevention & Treatment: Wash all clothes, bed lines, & towels in hot water the day after treatment and repeat in 1 week. Treat with the following: permethrin 5% cream (*Elimite*) or 1% *Nix* to entire body overnight then wash off **OR** crotamiton (*Eurax*) apply chin to feet, repeat in 24 hours, wash off in 48 hours **OR** ivermectin (*Stromectol*) 200 micrograms per kg orally **OR** 6% sulfur in petroleum cream applied overnight **OR** lindane lotion to body overnight then wash off [avoid if pregnancy or seizures].

Mites – Scrub Typhus (Tsutsugamushi)

Background:
- Scrub typhus is from a Rickettsia-like bacteria carried by chiggers
- Scrub describes the vegetation (between woods and clearings) than harbors the infected chigger (larvae of mites)
- Most cases occur in regions of eastern Asia, the southwest Pacific (Korea to Australia) and from Japan to India and Pakistan.

Features: Initially, a dark ulcer develops with lymph nodes (near the bite) and then generalized lymph node enlargement including an enlarged spleen and liver. Small blood vessels become inflamed (vasculitis) with development of a headache, muscle aches, injected conjunctiva (whites of eyes) 5-20 days after being infected. In 1/3, a red rash develops on the trunk. Brain involvement can occur.

Treatment: Treat with doxycycline or tetracycline. Alternately, use rifampin, azithromycin, or roxithromycin.

Mosquitoes

Mosquitoes transmit a large variety of illnesses around world (Table). See specific disease within guide for features & management and see table at bottom of page for mosquito bite prevention. See Dengue & Viral hemorrhagic fever pages 81-83, encephalitis pages 95, 96.

Disease/Virus[1]	Primary Disease Locations[1]
Dengue	Central/Sth Am, Africa, Asia, Southeast US
East. Equine V	Eastern/Gulf/South US, South America
Filariasis	Tropical regions Asia, Africa, South/Cent Am.
Malaria	See pages 99-101
Murray V	Australia, New Guinea
Japanese EN	Japan, China, Southeast Asia, India
Rift Valley fever	Sub-Saharan Africa
Ross River V	Australia, New Guinea, South Pacific
St. Louis EN	Central, West, Southern US
Valley EN	Australia, New Guinea
West Nile V	Africa, West Asia, Middle East, Europe, US
Yellow Fever	Africa, South America

[1] V – virus, EN – encephalitis, Am – America, US – United States

Mosquito Bite Prevention

- Limit outdoor time during dusk to dawn which is the most active time for mosquitoes.
- Wear loose fitting clothing & shoes/boots that cover most body.
- Remain in well screened areas as much as possible.
- Spray rooms at night with pyrethroid/pyrethrin flying insect spray and consider using mosquito coils or candles.
- Use mosquito bed nets treated with insecticides (e.g. permethrin, deltamethrin) at night.
- Use insect repellent with 30% DEET (N,N-diethyl-m-toluamide) on exposed skin for children > 2 months to 12 years old and 30-50% DEET for adults.
- Avoid use of DEET on mucous membranes (lips, eyes, nose) & wounds. 20% DEET lasts up to 4 hours, 25% -5 hours, 30% - 6-8 hours, while long acting preparations can last up to 12 hours. Reapply more frequently if lost due to sweating, swimming etc.
- Infants ≤ 2 months old, use carrier draped with mosquito net fitted tightly with elastic. DEET not recommended by AAP

Murine & Epidemic Typhus (see **Mites** for Scrub Typhus)
Background: Epidemic typhus is caused by Rickettsia transmitted
by human lice, while murine typhus is transmitted by rat fleas.
Features: Fever, headache, muscle aches, and nausea typically
develop 7-16 days after exposure. One third to ½ all patients
develop a rash that starts on the trunk and spreads to the arms and
legs. The rash is typically red and becomes pale with pressure
(blanches). Later non-blanching red areas, petechiae (bleeding), and
bruising develop. Lung involvement with cough, then pneumonia
can occur. Brain involvement with seizures, confusion, hearing loss,
and coma can develop. Red, irritated appearing conjunctiva are seen
in a minority.
Prevention & Treatment: Lice are killed by washing clothes and
sheets in hot water and drying > 5 minutes at > 131°C (55°C).
Doxycycline is the drug of choice. Alternatives include drugs that are
less well studied (azithromycin, rifampin).

Pediculosis (Lice)

Background:
- Lice are parasites that feed on human blood.
- Infestations (pediculosis) occur on the head, body & pubic region.
- Body lice can spread epidemic typhus and relapsing fever.
- Lice can spread by personal contact or via clothes & objects.

Features: Lice cause skin irritation, sores, and enlarged lymph
nodes. Head lice deposit eggs (nits) that attach within 3-4
millimeters of the scalp. Nits (lice eggs) fluoresce or shine in the
dark under ultraviolet light.
Prevention & Treatment: Individuals with body lice should destroy
their clothing. All clothing, sheets, and objects made of fabric (e.g.
stuffed animals) require washing in hot water with machine drying >
5 minutes at > 131°F (55°C). Remove nits using a comb (teeth 3-4
mm apart). Treat head lice with the following: benzyl alcohol
(Ulesfia) **OR** permethrin 1% (*Nix*) **OR** permethrin 5% cream
(*Elimite*) **OR** malathion (*Ovide*) **OR** lindane (See drug prescribing
info and precautions starting page 125) If body lice or treatment
failure: *Septra* DS or *Bactrim* 1 twice/day X 3 days repeat in 1 week,
(best if use with permethrin) **OR** ivermectin (*Stromectol*) 200
micrograms per kg X 1 – may repeat in 1 week

Scorpions

Background:

- Scorpions are found on all continents except Antarctica and are distributed between 50 degrees north and south of the equator.
- Most scorpions come out at night while during the day they hide under rocks, in burrows, or within plants.
- Scorpion size does not correlate with aggressiveness or potency.
- While most scorpions only cause local pain and inflammation, worldwide, there are 5000 deaths per year attributed to scorpions.
- Deaths from scorpion are only due to a few of the > 1000 known species of scorpions.
- Scorpions will fluoresce when exposed to ultraviolet light.

Important Venomous Scorpions

Class	Location	Important Symptoms[1,2]
Centruroides (bark scorpion)	US, Mexico, West Indies, South Am.	Pain, tingling, numbness, high BP/HR, confusion, abnormal eye movements
Leiurus (death stalker)	North Africa, Middle East	High BP/HR, high blood sugar, congestive heart failure
Tityus (devil scorpion)	Central/South Am. West Indies	Local pain, high BP/HR, congestive heart failure, pancreatitis
Androctonus (flat tailed scorpion)	North Africa, Middle East, Pakistan, India	Local pain, burning, sweating, seizures, confusion
Mesobuthus (red scorpion)	India	Local pain, paresthesias, high BP/HR, high blood sugar and high potassium

[1] BP – blood pressure, HR – heart rate,
[2] paresthesias – numbness or tingling

Scorpions

Features: Scorpions resemble miniature lobsters with small heads, segmented bodies, eight legs, two front claws, and a segmented tail ending in a venom containing sac with a stinger. They range in length from a few millimeters to > 15 centimeters. Most scorpion bites cause intense pain. Light tapping of the puncture site will often greatly increase the pain. Envenomation by poisonous scorpions usually causes cholinergic, adrenalin-like, neurologic symptoms or a combination of these features Initial symptoms can take up to 6 hours to manifest and are cholinergic in nature with the SLUDGE syndrome (Salivation, Lacrimation, Urine incontinence, Defecation, Gastrointestinal pain, and Emesis or vomiting). Subsequently, release of an adrenalin like substance (norepinephrine) causes an increased heart rate, blood pressure, temperature, elevated blood sugar, with depression of heart activity and congestive heart failure (fluid build-up in lungs). Other symptoms are neurologic and include confusion, agitation, an unsteady gait, restless muscles, and paralysis of breathing. Rarely, heart attacks and strokes can occur.

Prevention & Treatment: If working or traveling in an area with scorpions, shake out clothing and shoes/boots before dressing. Clothing, bedding, and camping gear also should be shaken out, inspected, and turned over since scorpions can hold onto these articles. Use gloves, long sleeved shirts, and closed toe shoes when exploring or working in scorpion habitats. Insecticides including organophosphates, pyrethrins, and some chlorinated hydrocarbons can kill scorpions. Insecticides also indirectly work by killing insects that constitute their food supply.

Most victims of scorpion envenomation only require local supportive care. If local signs and symptoms are present (local pain, paresthesias or tingling), observation for 4-6 hours may be all that is required. Local anesthetics can decrease pain from stings. Local wound care with cleansing and tetanus prophylaxis (See page 53) is required. If more than local toxicity is noted (e.g. cholinergic, adrenal-like, neurologic symptoms), hospital monitoring is required. Cholinergic symptoms can be reversed with intravenous atropine although this therapy is rarely required. Medications to treat hypertension, tachycardia, and therapy directed at congestive heart failure may be required.

Scorpion Sting Treatment

The use of antivenom is controversial as many experts feel it does not improve outcome, to work best it must be given within the 1st few hours after envenomation, it must be specific to the species that stings, and it is often not available. Local medical experts, wilderness medicine specialists, and toxicologists may aid in determining the need for antivenom.

Snakes

Background:
- Most snake bites are delivered by nonpoisonous species.
- Most poisonous snakes are classified into Viperidae (Crotalidae), Elapidae, Atractaspididae, and Colubridae (Table).
- There is no simple method for easily identifying poisonous snakes.
- Do not handle dead snakes as they can reflexly inject venom.
- Clinical features of venomous snake bites can include early local swelling with bleeding, early neurologic symptoms with altered mental status and weakness, or a combination of both.

Features: Most Viperidae have long hypodermic needle like fangs through which they inject venom. Their fangs can be long, curved, and hinged so that they can extend and retract their fangs into their mouth. Atractaspididae have long fangs whereby they stab their victims with a side swiping motion of a fang protruding from the corner of their mouth. Colubridae have fangs that are more posteriorly located and to envenomate (poison), these snakes often have to seize, hold onto, and chew victims. Many Elapidae (except large cobras) have short fangs and also must chew to completely envenomate. The fangs of African & Asian spitting cobras, and South African ringhal cobras can spray their venom more than 1 to 2 meter to blind victims.

Signs and symptoms of snake envenomation (poisoning) differ depending up on the type of snake involved. (Table) Fortunately, most snake bites are by nonvenomous species, while bites by venomous snakes do not inject venom in up to ½ of all cases. For venomous snakes, severity of envenomation is determined by the dose of venom injected (related to length of bite and size of snake), type composition of venom (related to species), the health and size of the victim, and the treatment rendered.

Select Venomous Snakes

Class	Examples	Poisoning Features
Atractasp-ididae	Asps Stiletto snakes Mole adders/vipers False vipers Natal black snake	Local pain, swelling, blistering, tissue necrosis, numbness and tingling. Severe poisoning can cause violent vomiting, salivation, weakness, and coma.
Viperidae (Crotalidae)	Rattlesnakes Adders Vipers Pit vipers Habu	Severe local swelling, local pain, local bruising, and bleeding. Skin and muscle necrosis occurs. Eventual bleeding from multiple sites with shock & kidney failure.
Elapidae	Brown snake Cobras Coral snake Krait, Mamba Mulga Sea snakes (painless bite) Taipan Tiger snake	Minimal local symptoms except cobras which can cause extensive swelling & blistering. Neurologic symptoms are prominent with vomiting, weak muscles (esp. eyes, mouth, then breathing). Dilated pupils. Onset of neurologic features can be 30 min to 12 hours.
Colubrids	Boomslang African twig snake African tree, vine, & twig snake	Local symptoms are usually minimal. Systemic symptoms include vomiting, abdominal pain, and headache. Spontaneous bleeding from gums, nose, GI tract and eventual kidney failure.

List of snakes is NOT all inclusive and many other types exist.

Prevention & Treatment:

Wear boots and coarse pants when walking. Be aware that after a natural disaster, snakes may be forced into unnatural areas (e.g. trees, and homes). Remain more than 2 snake body lengths from any identified snake. Do not pick up a dead snake as many can still inject venom even after death or it may be faking death.

Snake bite Treatment

• **Suspect a bite** occurred if there are a pair of puncture marks (or abrasions from chewing Elapidae), continued bleeding from wound, redness/swelling at site, severe pain at the site, vomiting, difficulty breathing, double vision or difficulty seeing, increased salivation or sweating, numbness or tingling in extremities/face
• **Kill & capture** the snake for identification ONLY if it is safe to do so
• **Keep the victim still**, supine & immobilized to slow venom spread
• **Splint** the bitten limb below the level of the heart
• **DO NOT** attempt unproven & harmful measures such as cutting, suctioning, applying ice, alcohol or aspirin
• **Pressure immobilization** may be useful for Australian Elapidae and some sea snakes. Apply pressure bandage from below bite upwards as far as possible to compress lymphatics on the affected limb. Apply as tight as for an ankle sprain without affecting pulses.
• **CAUTION:** if too tight, this can increase tissue damage
• **Rapidly transport** victim to nearest regional hospital with snake envenomation expertise and available antivenin/antivenom. Local experts will be most aware of venomous species in their area, and indications for antivenin/antivenom.

Spiders

Background:
- Spiders are found in all habitats except the sea.
- Of the > 30,000 worldwide species of species of spiders only a few dozen are venomous (poisonous).
- Toxicity from spiders can occur from injection of venom after biting or from direct contact from hairs that irritate the skin or mucous membranes (e.g. tarantulas).
- In North America, most necrotic or abscessed skin infections are due to local infection with bacteria (esp. methicillin resistant *Staphylococcus aureus*) and not due to spider bites.

Important Venomous Spiders

Spider Type	Common Location	Important Symptoms
Brown recluse or fiddleback	North/South Am., Mediterranean, Africa	Minimal pain with bite, tissue may die over days and weeks, systemic symptoms are rare
Australian Funnel web	Australia, South Pacific	Painful bite due to large fangs, rapid onset of severe symptoms with agitation, muscle twitching, confusion, ↑ blood pressure, pulmonary edema.
Hobo	North America, Europe, western Asia	Mostly local irritation, debate exists as to whether hobos cause brown recluse like necrosis.
Running/sac	Australia, Pacific, US, Europe, Africa	Painful local bite with irritation, and mild nausea/abdomen pain
Tarantula	US, Central/South Am, Caribbean, Africa, Australia Mediterranean	Painful, nontoxic bites, hairs are discharged from tarantula causing severe localized allergic type symptoms
Black Widow (*Redback spider*)	Widespread (*Australia*)	Minimal local symptoms, severe, muscle spasms, weakness, elevated BP, severe abdomen pain
Wolf	Widespread	Mostly localized irritation, and pain

Spiders can be divided into those that cause primarily local tissue injury/irritation, systemic (diffuse body) symptoms, or of both. Local trauma – most spiders cause no systemic symptoms with minimal localized trauma or irritation. This group includes jumping spiders, wolf spiders, orb weaving spiders, and many house dwelling (huntsman) and garden dwelling spiders. Slightly more local necrosis is caused by hobo, running, and sac spiders with occasional systemic symptoms including headache, malaise, and rarely hallucinations (hobo and grass spiders).

Brown recluse spiders are known for causing extensive tissue necrosis at the site of their bite. The recluse is small (1.5 centimeters) with a violin (fiddle) design on its back. The initial bite may or may not be painful with a small red ring that develops soon afterwards. Blistering with gray to purple skin discoloration can develop within 1-3 days followed by a painful ulcer occurring over the first week. Rarely, muscle damage with red blood cell and platelet breakdown occur leading to kidney damage. Most brown recluse bites heal without medical treatment.

Systemic symptoms - *Black widows* are spiders that are widespread often living in protected areas including buildings, wood piles, and in littered areas. The venom is a neurologic toxin that causes minimal local injury or toxicity. Victims initially complain of muscle pain and cramping that spreads to the entire body. Abdominal pain can be especially severe. Other findings can include salivation, sweating, tearing, tremors, heart rate abnormalities (high or low), high blood pressure, shock and coma. Most symptoms resolve within 2-3 days. The very young and old, and victims with cardiovascular disease are at increased risk for death or other complications. No deaths from black widow spider bites have been reported in the US in over a decade. The *Redback spider* is a relative of the black widow spider living in Australia. Symptoms are similar to those of black widow envenomation. *Australian funnel web spiders* are one of the most venomous spiders in the world. These spiders are usually 4 to 5 centimeters in length with 4-5 millimeter fangs that can penetrate fingernails and deep tissues making removal difficult. Fortunately, only 10-20% of bitten victims develop toxicity. The initial bite is extremely painful but local tissue damage is minimal. Systemic symptoms begin within 30 minutes of the bite with deaths (especially in children) reported within an hour of envenomation. Early symptoms include agitation, sweating, salivation, tearing, muscle spasms, abdomen pain. Blood pressure and heart rate can be elevated or depressed. Shock and muscle breakdown causing kidney failure are late findings. Pulmonary edema (fluid build-up in lungs) causing shortness of breath occurs in more than half of victims with severe envenomation. A minority of victims lose consciousness.

Spider Bite Prevention & Treatment:
Initial treatment for all bites includes local wound cleansing, and immobilization. If possible, safely kill & collect the spider for identification.

There is no <u>immediate</u> treatment other than local wound care needed for *brown recluse spider* bites. Antibiotics are used if there is any suspicion of localized infection. In many areas of the US, the majority of reported brown recluse spider bites are actually skin infections (with or without underlying abscess) due to methicillin resistant *Staphylococcus aureus* (MRSA). All abscesses require drainage, while MRSA can be treated with trimethoprim-sulfisoxazole, clindamycin, linezolid, or doxycycline. If severe, intravenous antibiotics may be needed. True brown recluse spider bites can cause chronic ulcers and scarring. Most experts recommend excising this tissue only after 6-8 weeks of localized wound care.

Spider bites due to either black widow spiders or Australian funnel web spiders may require more intensive therapy. Unproven measures to limit absorption of the venom include local application of ice, a loose compressive dressing (that does NOT obstruct venous or arterial blood flow), and immobilization of the extremity. Extraction devices are not proven to remove a significant amount of venom and may cause trauma increasing venom absorption. Patients with either of these bites require rapid transportation to a hospital. Airway support & blood pressure control may be required.

Muscle cramping and pain due to *black widow spider* bites can be treated with intravenous benzodiazepines (lorazepam, diazepam) and pain medications. Calcium injections to relieve cramping are not useful. Victims with severe symptoms, the very young and old, those with underlying heart disease, or vital sign abnormalities may require hospital admission for monitoring. Rarely, antivenom is used to treat severe systemic symptoms. Since black widows bites are rarely fatal, antivenom is reserved victims with severe symptoms/vital sign abnormalities and extremes of age or severe underlying disease. Antivenom is made from horse serum and can cause an immediate allergic reaction (up to 25% of cases) or delayed serum sickness (up to 75% of cases). Redback spider antivenom is available in Australia and administered intramuscularly indications similar to those for black widow antivenom (antivenin).

Immediate antivenom is indicated for Australian *funnel web envenomation* if any signs of envenomation occur. It is available in Australia & derived from rabbit serum. In Australia, the New South Wales Poison Center (61-2-9845-3111 or 131126 in Australia) can be contacted for advice. Fewer immediate and delayed symptoms occur from this antivenom compared to horse derived antivenom.

Ticks Diseases – Lyme Disease

Background:

- Lyme disease is due to a bacteria (spirochete) transmitted from ticks to humans.
- This disease is most common in North America and Europe although cases occur in North Africa and Asia.
- Less than ½ of all victims recall having a tick bite.

Features: The Early Localized Stage of Lyme disease typically begins 7-10 days (3-32 day range) after a tick bite. Initial symptoms include low grade fever, headache, and muscle aches. A typical rash (erythema migrans/EM) occurs in 60-90% of victims. EM is red, occurs at the site of the tick bite, is flat or slightly raised, and increases in size over several days with clearing or lightening of the central part of the rash. This rash is typically ≥ 5 centimeters (2 inches) in size and may grow to be much larger. Multiple skin lesions can be present. Within 4-6 weeks, untreated Lyme disease can progress to an Early Disseminated Stage that involves the neurologic system (headache/meningitis, weakness of face or eye muscles), the heart (inflammation, or slow heart rate), joint inflammation, and eye inflammation or visual loss. Late Stage disease occurs years later with chronic or recurrent arthritis (joint inflammation), weakness, confusion, or visual loss.

Prevention & Treatment: Tick bites can be prevented by wearing long sleeves and long pants while avoiding heavily forested areas. Application of DEET containing insect repellent can also prevent tick attachment and bites. Remove attached ticks (tick removal, page 74). A single 200 mg oral dose of doxycycline has been shown to prevent disease in persons bitten by ticks in endemic areas. Early local disease can be treated with doxycycline, amoxicillin, or cefuroxime for 21 days. More advanced or complicated disease may require up to 30 days of intravenous ceftriaxone or penicillin.

Tick Disease – Other Disorders

The list of diseases carried or caused by ticks is extensive and includes bacteria (Rocky Mountain Spotted fever, Rickettsial pox, Ehrlichiosis, Relapsing fever, Boutonneuse fever, tularemia), viruses (encephalitis, Crimean Congo hemorrhagic fever, Omsk hemorrhagic fever), parasites (Babesiosis), and toxins (tick paralysis).

Prevention & Treatment: Travelers should be aware that tick bites are not always apparent. Tick bites can be prevented by wearing long sleeves and long pants while avoiding walks in heavily forested areas. Application of DEET containing insect repellent can also prevent tick attachment and bites. Remove attached ticks. (Tick removal below)

Tick Removal

Wear gloves
If available, inject local anesthetic + epinephrine directly below tick
DO NOT apply petroleum jelly, alcohol, fingernail polish to tick[1]
DO NOT light a match to the underside of the tick[1]
Use blunt tweezers to grasp the tick as close as possible to the skin
Pull slowly & firmly directly away (perpendicular) from the skin
DO NOT squeeze tick & **DO NOT** rotate tweezers as pulling up
Cleanse the skin thoroughly after tick removal
Dispose of the tick via flushing down toilet or placing in alcohol
Thoroughly clean your hands after removal is complete
Consider a single dose of doxycycline if in area with Lyme disease

[1] This can cause regurgitation of spirochete (bacteria) & other organisms from the tick and introduction of disease into person bitten.

BURNS

Background:

- Smoke inhalation from fires in enclosed spaces can cause asphyxiation (low oxygen), carbon monoxide and cyanide toxicity.
- DO NOT apply ice to a burn as this can increase tissue injury.
- Electrical and chemical burns cause more damage than initially apparent on first evaluation.

Features: Burn depth is categorized as 1st degree (sunburn), 2nd degree (blisters, sensation intact), 3rd degree (white/charred skin, pain may be minimal, cannot see hair follicles) & 4th degree (involving bone, tendon, or muscle). While standard charts are more accurate, burned total body surface area (TBSA) can be estimated with a palm comprising 0.5% of a person's TBSA and a hand's entire palmar surface (with fingers) comprising slightly < 1% of a person's TBSA.

Major Burns Requiring Medical Evacuation & Hospital Admission	Burns involving ≥ 15% TBSA (≥ 10% for child) excluding 1st degree burns
	3rd degree burns ≥ 2% TBSA
	Significant chemical/electrical burns
	Respiratory tract burns
	Associated major trauma
	Carbon monoxide/cyanide toxicity
	Burns that encircle an extremity

Prevention & Treatment: Remove constricting clothing or jewelry as soon as possible. Remove chemicals by brushing or rinsing the area with clean water. DO NOT try to neutralize chemicals (e.g. apply acid to base). *Major burns* (table) require admission and are best managed at a hospital. Oxygen, intravenous fluids, and specialized wound care are required to prevent shock, pneumonia, infection, tissue loss, and organ failure. Do not apply cold water to large areas for comfort control as this can lower a victim's temperature. *Minor 2nd & 3rd degree burns* can be treated with local measures. Cool water (NOT ice) can be applied to small areas to decrease swelling and pain. Cleanse wounds with soap and water, remove dead tissue, leave blisters intact, apply topical antibiotics to burns that are 2nd degree or greater and cover with gauze. *1st degree Sunburn or Equivalent* can be treated with oral anti-inflammatory agents (ibuprofen) or a short course of oral steroids. Topical aloe vera may provide additional anti-inflammatory effects.

CARDIAC EMERGENCIES
Cardiac Arrest – General Approach for Non-professionals

- All travelers should take a course in CPR (cardiopulmonary resuscitation) and basic life support. The information listed is only relayed to serve as a reminder to concepts already learned.
- Because it is difficult for the untrained to assess whether a pulse is present, check for responsiveness to shaking & loud talking, chest movement, and air moving through a victim's mouth.
- Chest compressions are performed to deliver blood to vital organs as a stop gap while waiting for advanced life support. Ventilations, in adults, are less important & can be deferred for 1st few minutes.
- Guidelines and algorithms spend excess effort relaying unproven specific time intervals, depth of chest compressions, and frequency of ventilation and chest compressions (CPR table).
- DO NOT Spend excess time trying to meet number goals in CPR chart. More importantly (1) identify victims not breathing or without a pulse, (2) open an airway and assist breathing (3) apply an automated external defibrillator to non-breathing unresponsive victims and (4) quickly begin chest compressions to victims without a pulse until advanced life support is available.

Cardiopulmonary Resuscitation (CPR) Maneuvers, Techniques

Maneuver	Infant < 1 year	Child (1-8 years)	> 8years
Airway open	Jaw lift if trauma, otherwise head tilt & chin lift		
Breathing			
Initial	Give initial 2 breaths - enough to cause chest to rise		
No CPR	12-20/minute	12-20/minute	10-12/minute
CPR	8-10/minute	8-10/minute	8-10/minute
Circulation			
Compress location	Low ½ sternum	Low ½ sternum	Low ½ sternum
Compress with	Hands/thumbs encircle chest	Heel of one hand	Heel of one hand
Depth	One third to one half depth of chest		1.5 – 2 inches
Rate[1]	100/minute	100/minute	100/minute
Ratio[2]	15:2	15:2	30:2

[1]Total #of events (compressions + breaths, [2]Ratio for 2 person CPR
Foreign body obstruction < 1 year, apply back blows or chest thrusts, if older abdominal thrust (Heimlich) 1st, then chest thrust/back blow

Cardiac Arrest – Adults & Adolescent after Puberty[1]

No Movement or Response or only minimal Gasping

↓

Call 911 (or Ambulance if no 911 service) AND Obtain defibrillator (e.g. AED[2]) if available

↓

Check Pulse[3] for 10 seconds	→ *Definite* → *Pulse*	• Give **1 breath** every 5 to 6 seconds

↓ *No pulse*

• Check pulse every 2 minutes

• Give **30 Compressions & 2 Breaths**[4]. Compress ≥ 100/minute. • Minimize interruptions in compressions • 2 rescuers: switch ventilation/compression roles every 2 minutes

↓ Once AED available

Check for shockable rhythm with AED[2] Place & Turn on AED, then follow AED instructions

↙ shockable   ↘ not shockable

Give 1 shock, Resume CPR immediately for 2 minutes	Resume CPR immediately for 2 minutes, check rhythm with AED every 2 minutes. Continue until advanced life support (ambulance arrives)

[1] Puberty = axilla/armpit hair in males, breast development females.

[2] AED – Automatic External Defibrillator. An AED should only be placed on unresponsive or pulseless individuals. First, turn ON the AED. Then follow the computer generated voice instructions. It will prompt you to place adhesive electrode pads on a victim's bare chest. It will then analyze the heart rhythm. If the machine determines that a rhythm is present that might respond to shocking, it will charge itself and then tell you to press a button that delivers a shock. NEVER touch the victim during shocking or during rhythm analysis.

[3] Shaded instructions are only for medical professionals. Skip this step if non-trained, non-medical professional.

[4] Compressions without breaths may be appropriate for lay people to perform in prehospital setting in cardiac arrest victims.

Cardiac Arrest – Infants & Children up to Puberty[1]
Basic Resuscitation for Non-Professional Bystanders

Unresponsive, Not breathing, or only minimal Gasping
If 2nd person available, have them call 911 & get AED[2]
- Lone rescuer (non-professional) go to **un**shaded box[3]
- Lone rescuer (medical professional) – see shaded boxes

Check Pulse for 10 seconds *(brachial/inner arm in infant & femoral groin in child)*	→ *Definite Pulse*	Give **1 breath** every 3 seconds, Compress if HR < 60 per minute despite adequate oxygenation & ventilations, Check pulse every 2 minutes

↓ *No pulse*

- **Single Rescuer** - Give **30 Compressions & 2 Breaths**
- **2 Rescuers** - **Compress and Breathe at 15:2 ratio**
- Compress at ≥ 100/minute, allow recoil after each compression
- Minimize compression interruptions & avoid excess ventilation
- Rescuers - switch ventilation/compression roles every 2 minutes

↓

Single rescuer – after 2 minutes, call 911 and get AED if available

↓

Check for shockable rhythm with AED
Place & Turn on AED, then follow AED instructions

↙ shockable   ↘ not shockable

Give 1 shock, resume CPR immediately for 2 minutes	Resume CPR immediately for 2 minutes, check rhythm with AED every 2 minutes, Continue until ambulance or help arrives.

[1] Puberty = axilla/armpit hair in males, breast development females.
[2] AED – Automatic External Defibrillator. AED with pediatric attenuator is preferred for children < 8 years old although those without a dose attenuator may be used if they are the only choice.
[3] Lone healthcare providers suspicious of cardiac event (e.g. sudden collapse during athletic event) may opt to immediately get AED instead of beginning CPR. However, Lone NON-healthcare professionals should begin compressions immediately.

HYPOTHERMIA

Background:

- Hypothermia can be mild (core temperature > 34-35°C/93°F), moderate (30-34°C/86-93°F) or severe (< 30°C/< 86°F).
- Oral temperatures are unreliable if more than mild hypothermia.
- The body no longer can shiver to increase body temperature at temperatures below 31°C/88°F.
- Multiple factors including age extremes (very young & old), neurologic disorders, endocrine disease (e.g. diabetes), immersion in water, cardiovascular disease, drugs and toxins (e.g. alcohol), and trauma predispose travelers to developing hypothermia.

Clinical Features of Hypothermia

Severity	*Features*
Mild (> 34-35°C 93-95°F)	• Shivering is present, metabolism increases • Slurred speech, relatively normal blood pressure and respirations
Moderate (30-34°C 86-93°F)	• Loss of coordination (esp. with walking) • Altered mental status, confusion • Shivering disappears • Irregular and skipped heart beat
Severe (< 30°C < 86°F)	• Pupils dilate • ↓ in heart rate, blood pressure & respirations with eventual cardiac standstill • progressive loss of consciousness • Reflexes are delayed, then disappear

Prevention & Treatment:

Afterdrop: Once a moderately or severely hypothermic victim is removed from the cold, their core temperature may continue to drop. This "afterdrop" is due to mixing of the cooler peripheral blood with warmer core blood. This effect also may cause life-threatening heart rhythms during rewarming in severely hypothermic victims treated with external rewarming techniques. For this reason, external rewarming of severely hypothermic victims is NOT recommended. Excess movement or vigorously handling of severely hypothermic victims also can contribute to afterdrop and is discouraged.

Hypothermia Management

Remove wet clothing and assist ventilation if needed. Use a low reading rectal thermometer and NOT a tympanic or oral thermometer to determine a hypothermic victim's temperature.

Severity	Management
Mild (> 34-35°C/93-95°F)	• Passive external rewarming –Warm blankets or other surface measures
Moderate (30-34°C/86-93°F)	• Active external rewarming requires hospitalization with warmed oxygen & warm intravenous fluids. • Electric external warming blankets can be used (e.g. Bair Hugger)
Severe (< 30°C/< 86°F)	• External rewarming techniques have the potential to cause a significant temperature "afterdrop" (page 79) and are not recommended until well after active internal rewarming started • Active internal rewarming in an intensive care unit is recommended. This can involve infusion of saline around lungs, into peritoneum (abdominal cavity), bladder, or cardiopulmonary bypass.

FROSTBITE

Frostbite occurs when tissues freeze with ice crystal formation. High altitude, age extremes, water, poor nutrition, localized infection, nicotine use, prior cold injury, and vascular disease are risk factors. Extremities, face, and ears are the most common sites. ¾ of patients report numbness and clumsiness. Address life-threats 1st while administering fluids (if possible) & pain medications. Initially manage by removing constricting jewelry and wet clothing while insulating and immobilizing affected areas. DO NOT apply dry heat to gradually thaw. DO NOT rub area to rewarm. If no evacuation is possible, rapid field rewarming in water at 40-42°C (some recommend 35-40°C) is one option. However, DO NOT rewarm when there is a potential for refreezing as this will worsen the injury. Patients are treated as if they have a deep burn with surgery reserved for tissue that is obviously dead (often 1-3 months after injury).

DENGUE

Background:

- Worldwide, up to 100 million cases of Dengue occur per year with ½ million yearly cases of Dengue Hemorrhagic Fever (DHF).
- 20-30% of DHF cases develop shock Dengue Shock Syndrome
- Dengue is most commonly found in Central & South America, the Caribbean, Africa, Southeast Asia, India, and the western Pacific.
- Prior infection with one of the 4 types of dengue does not protect from developing dengue from the other serotypes.

Features: Dengue usually begins 3-14 days after a mosquito bite. Many children often have minimal fever or no symptoms. Adults and older children frequently have a fever > 30°C (102.2°F) with more extensive symptoms (Table). Some develop rapid deterioration after a few days of mild symptoms with the development of severe bleeding (Dengue Hemorrhagic Fever/DHF) or shock (Dengue Shock Syndrome). Children < 15 years old account for 90% of DHF cases possibly due to their more fragile capillaries.

Features of Dengue (D) & Dengue Hemorrhagic Fever (DHF)

Organ	Features
Abdomen (esp. in DHF)	• Abdomen pain, vomiting, gastrointestinal bleeding, liver inflammation/enlargement
Blood	• Low platelets, low hemoglobin [Hb] (anemia) from bleeding or high Hb due to dehydration.
Bones	• Severe bone pain is common in D (*break bone fever*), but less common in DHF
Brain	• Severe headache is common to D and DHF • Irritability, encephalitis, seizures, depression occur in both but are more common in DHF • DHF can cause brain swelling and bleeding
Skin (*more extensive bleed in DHF*)	• Transient red, flat rash may appear on day 1-2 • Bruising/petechiae occur as fever disappears • A positive "tourniquet test" in DHF > Dengue[1]
Other sites	• Nontender lymph nodes in neck, arms, & groin • Fluid leak into lungs (pulmonary edema)

[1]To perform this test inflate a blood pressure (BP) cuff on the upper arm and hold the BP between the diastolic (lower number) and systolic (upper number) BP. Positive test; > 20 petechiae (bleeding spots) over one square inch (2.2 centimeter) area on the forearm.

Dengue Prevention & Treatment: When traveling to endemic areas, mosquito preventative measures are required (See page 63). No vaccines are currently available for preventing Dengue.

Travelers with mild dengue symptoms, who are healthy with no underlying disease, and no suspicion of DHF or DSS do not require hospitalization. Treatment is symptomatic with avoidance of medicines that affect platelets (no aspirin or anti-inflammatory agents). If severe symptoms are present or there is suspicion of DHF or DSS, hospitalization will be required often in an intensive care unit setting. Treatment consists of blood pressure, heart, and breathing support. Blood products may be necessary. There are no medications effective against this virus.

OTHER VIRAL HEMORRHAGIC FEVERS (VHF)

Multiple other viruses can cause a potential lethal disease with fever, bleeding from mucous membranes and the gastrointestinal tract, along with swelling and a low blood pressure. (Table)

Background & Facts:

- Transmission occurs from bites (mosquitoes, ticks), aerosolized excrement (rodents) & direct contact with infected persons or livestock. Respiratory droplets may transmit some VHFs.
- Strict isolation is required with care-takers needing face (HEPA filter), hand, and body protection.
- A biologic terror attack should be considered if a VHF outbreak occurs in an uncommon (non-endemic) area or within a large number of military personnel.
- Vaccines are available for yellow fever, Argentine HF (may be effective vs. Bolivian HF), Rift Valley fever, and hanta virus strains causing renal failure.

Features: Most symptoms related to hemorrhagic fevers are due to VHFs attacking blood vessels and causing fluid leakage. Victims often have skin flushing, bleeding under the skin (petechiae and bruising), fever, swelling, and muscle aches. Later bleeding occurs from all membranes with a drop in blood pressure and shock. Bleeding is especially prominent in Ebola, Marburg, Crimean-Congo HF, and the rodent transmitted HFs. Edema (swelling) is especially prominent in Lassa fever. Blood cells break down with failure of the brain, lungs, with death 10% (dengue HF) to 90% (Ebola, Marburg).

Diseases Causing Viral Hemorrhagic Fever

Disease[1]	Common Location	Usual Vector	Onset after Exposure
Argentine (Junin) HF	South America	Rodents	1-2 weeks
Bolivian (Machupo) HF	South America	Rodents	1-2 weeks
Brazilian (Sabia) HF	South America	Rodents	1-2 weeks
Crimean-Congo HF	Europe, Asia, Africa	Tick	3-12 days
Dengue (See pages 81-83 for detail)	Americas, Africa, Asia	Mosquito	3-5 days[2]
Ebola	Africa	Unknown	3-16 days
Hantavirus HF or pulmonary syndrome	Worldwide	Rodent	1-5 weeks
Lassa fever	Africa	Rodent	5-16 days
Marburg	Africa	Unknown	3-16 days
Rift Valley fever	Africa	Mosquito	2-5 days
Venezuelan HF	South America	Rodent	1-2 weeks
Yellow fever (See page 124 for detail)	Tropical Africa, South America	Mosquito	3-6 days

[1] HF – hemorrhagic fever, [2] unknown onset for Dengue HF

Prevention & Treatment: Vaccines are available for yellow fever (See page 124), Argentine HF (which may be effective vs. Bolivian HF), Rift Valley fever, and hanta virus strains causing renal failure. When traveling to endemic areas, mosquito preventative measures are required (page 63). Importantly, no dead animals (or humans) should be handled. If victims within a party developed suspected VHF, barrier precautions should be taken (HEPA mask, gloves, barrier precautions) and contact should be limited.

All victims with suspected VHF require hospital admission and strict barrier precautions to prevent disease transmission. For most VHF, treatment consists of blood pressure and pulmonary support. Blood products may be necessary. Ribavirin is the only effective drug for treating Lassa fever and Hantavirus Hemorrhagic Fever with Renal Syndrome. Some experts also recommend this agent for South American HFs (Argentina, Bolivian, Brazilian, Venezuelan), Rift Valley Fever, and Crimean-Congo HF.

FISH & SHELLFISH INGESTED TOXINS

Background:
- Most fish related toxins are not eradicated with cooking.
- Symptoms may be due to inherent toxins or improper fish storage (scromboid) or contamination with dinoflagellates (plankton).

Features:

Scromboid occurs after eating improperly stored or refrigerated (< 40°F or 4.4°C is required) dark meat fish (tuna, mackerel, or mahi-mahi). Symptoms are due to histamine produced on the surface of improperly stored fish. Complaints include facial flushing, rash, itching, abdomen pain, diarrhea and a metallic taste. Tongue swelling, blurred vision, and respiratory distress can occur.

Ciguatera poisoning occurs after ingestion of predatory reef fish (barracuda, grouper, snapper, shark) with high concentrations of a dinoflagellate, *Gambierdiscus toxicus*. Vomiting, abdominal pain, and diarrhea, occur within the 1st few hours. Later weakness, tingling, itching, tooth pain, a loose teeth feeling, and a reversal of hot/cold sensation occurs. Within 1-3 days, a low blood pressure, a low heart rate, or abnormal heart rhythm can occur.

Paralytic Shellfish Poisoning (PSP) occurs after eating bivalve shellfish (clams, oysters, scallops, mussels) contaminated by dinoflagellates (*Alexandrium tamarense*) from "red tides". Headache, numbness, muscle weakness & breathing difficulty occur.

Puffer fish or fugu contain a neurologic toxin or tetrodotoxin. The flesh of this fish is a delicacy in Japan. Only trained and certified chefs should prepare this dish. Rarely, this toxin is found in the California newt, blue ringed octopus, and parrot fish. Symptoms begin 15 minutes to several hours after ingestion. Initially, tingling and numbness occur, followed by excess saliva, vomiting, diarrhea, and abdomen pain. Eventually weakness (esp. of breathing muscles), paralysis, and a drop in blood pressure, heart rate and death occur.

Prevention & Treatment: Cooking does not prevent poisoning from any of the listed toxins although experts recommend removing the viscera and gonads of shellfish and discarding the cooking liquid to reduce the risk of PSP. Scromboid can be alleviated by administering antihistamines (diphenhydramine/*Benadryl*). For the other toxins, treatment involves hospitalization with support of respirations, blood pressure, and heart rate.

HEPATITIS A

Background:
- Hepatitis A is the commonest vaccine preventable travel infection.
- This disease is spread via contaminated food.
- Many adults from developed countries have an acquired immunity.

Features: Symptom onset is 2-6 weeks after exposure. Symptoms include fatigue, loss of appetite, vomiting. Jaundice (yellow skin, eyes), dark urine, pale stools and abdomen pain from a big liver. Most recover without any long term effects. Rare deaths are reported (esp. if underlying liver disease or aged > 50 years).

Prevention & Treatment: Adherence to food and beverage precautions (see traveler's diarrhea) can prevent this disease. A hepatitis A (or A + B combination) vaccine is recommended for all travelers not already immune & older than 1 year (Canada, Europe) or older than 2 years (United States recommendation). It is given at least 2 weeks before travel with a booster at 6-12 months. For traveler's leaving in < 1-2 weeks to endemic hepatitis A areas, most experts feel that vaccine alone can prevent most illness. Treatment includes hydration, nausea/vomiting medications (e.g. ondansetron [*Zofran*], promethazine [*Phenergan*]) and avoiding products metabolized by the liver like acetaminophen/paracetamol & alcohol.

LEPTOSPIROSIS

Background:
- Leptospirosis is transmitted via urine of infected animals and is carried in soil and water (esp. common during flooding).
- The organism usually enters via mucous membranes & skin.

Features: Symptoms begin within 7-12 days of exposure. Initial symptoms include fever, chills, muscle aches, diarrhea, and reddening of the whites of the eyes (conjunctiva). After 4-7 days, the fever often resolves. A 2nd stage starts 1-2 days later with headache due to meningitis, occasional jaundice (yellow skin/eyes) & an enlarged spleen. Inflammation can occur within the eye, the heart, the skin (bruising) and kidneys with the potential for kidney failure.

Prevention & Treatment: Avoid swimming in freshwater contaminated by livestock or wildlife urine. Doxycycline 200 mg once per week can prevent disease if at high risk. Treatment consists of doxycycline, penicillin, amoxicillin, or cephalosporins X 7 days.

OTHER FOOD RELATED TOXINS & INFECTIONS
Botulism (*Clostridium botulinum*)
Background:
- Botulism occurs from a bacterial toxin found in soil and occasionally home canned foods.
- Infants can directly ingest bacterial spores (esp. contaminated honey) with bacteria directly producing the toxin in their bodies.

Features: Symptoms include the 4Ds (dry mouth, double vision, difficulty swallowing, difficulty talking). Paralysis of arms, legs, and respiratory muscles can occur. Infants may present with constipation, a weak cry and loss of tone.

Prevention & Treatment: Avoid home canned foods. Treatment consists of airway, breathing, & blood pressure support. The Centers for Disease Control has antitoxin that may reverse symptoms.

Brucellosis
Background:
- Brucellosis is a bacteria transmitted by infected food products (esp. unpasteurized milk and cheese) or via inhalation.
- Brucellosis most commonly occurs in locations where the handling of animals and dairy products is non-hygenic (the Middle East, the Mediterranean, China, India, Peru, and Mexico).

Features: The onset of symptoms can range from 1 to 8 weeks after exposure. The most frequent symptoms include relapsing fevers, chronic fatigue, and joint & back pain. In fewer cases, headache, depression, and irritability occur. Meningitis manifests as severe headache, altered mental status, neck pain or stiffness, or seizures. Abdomen pain with liver & spleen enlargement or abscess formation can occur. Rarely, endocarditis (heart valve) infections occur.

Prevention & Treatment: Brucellosis can be prevented by not handling animal products and pasteurizing all milk products. Disease is treated with doxycycline or with (streptomycin or rifampin). Ciprofloxacin (*Cipro*) also may be effective.

Staphylococcus aureus toxins cause nausea and vomiting within 6 hours of ingesting contaminated food (e.g. mayonnaise, eggs, confections, potato salad). Symptoms last < 1 to 2 days and treatment consists of vomiting medications and hydration.

TRAVELER's DIARRHEA
Background:

- *Traveler's diarrhea* (TD) is defined as ≥ 3 stools in 24 hours with ≥ 1 of the following: cramps, abdomen pain, vomiting, or fever.
- *Dysentery* is defined as the presence of visible blood in the stool.
- Enterotoxigenic Escherichia coli (ETEC) is a common cause of traveler's diarrhea in Central America, Africa and the Middle East.

Causes & Features of Traveler's Diarrhea

Agent	Onset	Sources	Symptoms
Campylobacter jejuni	2-5 days (after exposure)	Raw poultry, unpasteurized milk, water	Diarrhea, cramps, vomiting
Entamoeba histolytica (amebiasis)	2-4 weeks or longer	Water or food contaminated with feces	Gradual onset eventually bloody, liver abscess
Enterotoxigenic *E. coli*	1-3 days	Water or food contaminated with feces	Watery diarrhea, cramps, vomiting
Giardia	1-2 weeks or longer	Contaminated water supply, also in streams contaminated by animals	Gradual onset chronic diarrhea, bloating, gas, belching, weight loss
Salmonella	1-3 days	Eggs, poultry, unpasterurized milk, reptiles	Diarrhea, fever, abdomen pain,
Shigella	1-2 days	Water of food contaminated with feces	Diarrhea (often bloody), fever, abdomen pain
Vibrio cholera & non-cholera	12 hours – 7 days	Seafood and occasionally vegetables	Profuse watery diarrhea, no fever with cholera

Amebiasis, Salmonella, Shigella, and Vibrio have a propensity to cause blood borne infection and spread to other sites within the body.

Prevention & Treatment: The most important method for preventing traveler's diarrhea (TD) is to avoid unprepared food and drinks (See page 12, 13). Foods should be freshly cooked, served hot, and not diluted with water. Drinks should be bottled and sealed. The primary agent recommended for TD prevention is bismuth subsalicylate. Adults take 2 ounces or 2 tablets 4 times per day upon arrival at destination until home for 2 days. Since this agent contains aspirin, do not use it if you are taking blood thinners, already on aspirin products or anti-inflammatory agents, or cannot take high dose aspirin products. While antibiotics can prevent TD, many experts recommend against their use due to increasing resistance, multiple side effects, and their ability to only diminish symptoms only a few days once symptoms begin. Antibiotics (table) can be used to prevent TD & are reserved for high risk patients (i.e. immunocompromised) taking trips for short time. In Europe, an oral cholera vaccine (*Dukoral*) is available that is between 50 and 85% effective. It also may have some effect against enterotoxigenic *Escherichia coli*. In the US, no vaccine is available and the Center for Disease Control (CDC) does not recommend its use for most.

Treatment of Traveler's Diarrhea (TD)

Rehydration	Rehydrate with balanced electrolyte solutions.
Bismuth Subsalicylate	In adults, take 1 ounce or 2 tablets every 30 minutes for 8 doses. See caution above.
Anti-motility Agents	Loperamide or diphenoxylate can decrease diarrhea. Do not use if fever, bloody diarrhea, or severe vomiting.
Antibiotics *(Do not use at same time as Bismuth Subsalicylate)*	Organism unknown (adults): azithromycin (*Zithromax*) **OR** ciprofloxacin (*Cipro*) **OR** levofloxacin (*Levaquin)* **OR** rifaximin (*Xifaxan*) for 3 days. Organism known (adults): *Salmonella, Shigella, Campylobacter, E.coli,* - above unknown regimen. *Vibrio cholera* – azithromycin 1 g X 1 **OR** doxycycline 300 mg X 1 **OR** *Septra* DS 3 days; Giardia or *Entamoeba histolytica* – metronidazole (*Flagyl),* or tinidazole (*Tindamax*) with 2nd agent if severe disease or complications.

Typhoid Fever (Enteric fever)

Background:
- Typhoid fever is a disease cause by a strain of Salmonella (*Salmonella typhi* or *Salmonella paratyphi* A) which usually occurs following ingestion of food or water contaminated by a typhoid carrier.
- Worldwide, there are over 21 million cases reported per year.
- Most cases are contracted in Asia (esp. India), Africa, and Latin America. In Indonesia & New Guinea this is one of the 5 most common causes of death.

Features: Symptoms usually begin 1-3 weeks after exposure. Some develop abdominal pain and diarrhea in the disease course. For most, fever is the first sign of disease and persists for 2-3 weeks. Headache, muscle pain, weakness are common. Bacteria invade the lymphatic system, causing enlarged lymph nodes, and an enlarged liver and spleen. An altered mental status and seizures can occur. Heart rate may be relatively slow for a patient's level of fever. A minority of patients has small 2-4 mm red spots on their trunk and abdomen (rose spots). Intestinal bleeding or perforation can occur late in the disease and may be life-threatening.

Prevention & Treatment: The most important step in preventing typhoid fever is to only eat and drink food/beverages that have been appropriately cooked, prepared, and stored (page 12-13). An injectable and a live attenuated oral vaccine are available with each only demonstrating 70% effectiveness. The live vaccine is contraindicated in pregnancy and in those with a weakened immune system.

Resistance to antibiotics has limited the choice of available agents for treating typhoid fever. Ciprofloxacin is the drug of choice for non-resistant strains. For travelers from regions (India, Bangladesh, Pakistan, Vietnam) with high resistance, ceftriaxone (*Rocephin*) is recommended. A subset of patients may benefit from intravenous corticosteroid administration.

Following resolution of disease, 2-5% of victims develop a chronic carrier state with organisms often residing within the gallbladder. This may cause a relapse in a subset of patients.

OVERVIEW OF DIVING INJURIES

Dysbarism is defined as disease caused by a change in environmental pressure and is most commonly encountered in the setting of diving in water (e.g. SCUBA diving). Changes in pressure can cause trauma (barotrauma) during descent, during a dive, during ascent, or in a delayed fashion after ascent. Diseases placing travelers at risk include asthma, emphysema (COPD), infections & allergies (increased mucosal inflammation, plugging), structural obstruction (airway, sinus, ears, lungs), and panic disorders (too rapid ascent).

The **Diver's Alert Network (DAN)** has contact information for diving emergencies at many international sites. Visit the website and record contact information for your destination prior to travel.

DAN website	www.diversalertnetwork.org/
DAN phone numbers (see website for more specific contacts)	
Asia-Pacific (Australia +)[1]	In Australia: 1-800-088-200 Outside Australia: 62-8-8212-9242
Europe	39-06-4211-8685
Japan, Northeast Asia-Pacific	81-3-3812-4999
Malaysia	05-930-4114
Latin America	1-919-684-9111
North America(United States)	1-919-684-8111 or 1-919-684-4DAN
Philippines	02-815-9911
South Africa (SA)	In SA: 0800-020111 Outside SA: 27-11-254-1112

[1] Australia + New Zealand, Indonesia, Southeast Asia, China, Taiwan

BAROTRAUMA of ASCENT
Arterial Gas Embolism

Background:

- After drowning, arterial gas embolism (AGE) also called dysbaric air embolism is the most common cause of death in sport divers.
- AGE occurs when air bubbles cross the alveoli in the lungs into the circulation & throughout the body (especially heart & brain)
- Assume any diver that passes out while surfacing or *within 10 minutes of surfacing* has arterial gas embolism.

Features: Air Gas Emboli (AGE) can travel to the heart causing cardiac arrest, abnormal heart rhythms, and heart attacks. When bubbles enter the arteries to the brain, stroke like symptoms, seizures, an altered mental status, and headaches can occur. Chest pain, bloody cough, and shortness of breath can be prominent.

Prevention & Management: AGE can be prevented by strictly adhering to dive tables/dive computers and ascending at an appropriate rate. Exhaling normally during ascent also will decrease the possibility of developing AGE. All divers with symptoms suggestive of AGE require treatment even if symptoms resolve. Previously, it was recommended that victims be tilted head down with their feet elevated (Trendelenburg). However, this can increase brain edema, and worsen lung mechanics and is no longer recommended. Importantly, during air evacuation, cabin pressures should be maintained at sea level if possible. High flow oxygen can lessen symptoms. Definitive treatment involves compression to a treatment depth (usually 60 feet), and breathing high percentage oxygen at a partial pressure of 2.8 to 3 atmospheres. See DAN contacts for nearest compression chamber, page 90.

Decompression Sickness (DCS)

Background:

- DCS is also known as the bends, chokes, staggers, and niggles.
- DCS occurs when gas dissolved in the bloodstream (usually nitrogen) forms bubbles in the blood and tissues during ascent.
- Risk factors for DCS include prolonged, deep dives, diving at higher altitudes (e.g. lakes), advanced age, obesity, fatigue, colder water, exertion, dehydration, fever, and flying after diving.
- Any symptom that starts more than 10 minutes after a dive is DCS until proven otherwise.

Features: Type I Decompression Sickness (DCS) causes mild pain that often resolves within 10 minutes of ascent with itching/burning of the skin and a mottled or violet appearing rash. Swelling of extremities may occur from obstruction of lymphatic vessels. Most victims complain of deep aching pain in their joints or tendons that progressively worsens over time. In some cases, inflating a blood pressure cuff placed on the affected joint to 150-200 mm Hg will relieve the pain and confirm the presence or DCS.

Type II DCS causes chest/lung symptoms ("chokes"), neurologic symptoms, and shock. Pain is less common in type II DCS (only 1/3 of cases). Symptoms can occur immediately or up to 24-48 hours after diving. Chest complaints include shortness of breath, chest pain, cough, and increased respirations. Neurologic symptoms can include signs of spinal cord injury (incontinence or inability to hold urine or stool, back pain with lower extremity paralysis), or stroke (visual loss, confusion, weakness and headache). Importantly, arterial gas emboli can cause symptoms of brain injury, but not spinal cord injury. Shock can manifest as loss of consciousness, blacking out, sweating, or weakness.

Prevention & Treatment: DCS can be prevented by adhering to dive tables/ computers and ascending at an appropriate rate. Avoid risk factors (See Background). Previously, it was recommended that victims be placed in a head down tilted angle with their feet elevated (Trendelenburg). This position can increase brain edema & worsen lung mechanics & is no longer recommended. Administer 100% oxygen if available. Perform recompression as soon as possible in a hyperbaric chamber is the only definitive treatment (See DAN contacts, page 90). If air travel is required, transport at a low altitude (< 1000 feet or < 300 meters). Hyperbaric experts should guide specific therapy during recompression.

Pulmonary Over-Pressurization Syndrome/POPS
Background:
- Pulmonary Over-pressurization Syndrome (POPS) is also called pulmonary barotrauma of ascent or "burst lung".
- POPS occurs from expansion of gas trapped in the lungs with rupture of the alveoli and spread of air throughout the chest cavity.
- The greatest risk of POPS is from water < 10 feet salt water [fsw].
- Deaths from POPS have occurred in depths as shallow as 4 feet.

Features: Most (but not all) divers with POPS have a history of an uncontrolled rapid ascent to the surface. Air released from POPS can cause arterial gas emboli (AGE). Released air also can cause a collapsed lung which can lead to chest pain, shortness of breath or compression of the blood vessels returning to the heart with resulting low blood pressure (shock) and a loss of consciousness. Air bubbles can occasionally be felt under the skin.

Prevention & Management. A slow controlled ascent can prevent POPS. For diagnosis and treatment of suspected AGE see page 90-91. A significant collapsed lung may required a tube to decompress the pressure on the lung (chest tube).

Alternobaric Vertigo (ABV)

ABV is due to the inability to equalize middle ear pressures during ascent. This disorder is more common with allergies or inflamed mucosa of the Eustachian tubes (draining ears to back of throat). Symptoms can include a spinning sensation (vertigo) with nausea and vomiting. They may be severe enough to cause a diver to panic and rapidly ascend leading to more serious consequences of rapid ascent (AGE, DCS, POPS). After ascent, bed rest, suspension of diving, antihistamines, and decongestants may be of benefit.

BAROTRAUMA of DESCENT (Squeeze)
Background:
- Barotrauma of descent is due to compression of gas in enclosed spaces (e.g. ear, sinuses) during underwater descent.
- Increased pressure can cause bleeding, rupture of tissues, or formation of holes or fistulas (e.g. ruptured ear drum).

Features: The most common type of ear barotrauma is middle ear squeeze (barotitis media) which occurs due to failure of the middle ear and environmental pressures to equalize. Predisposing factors include a blocked Eustachian tube (ear to posterior pharynx connection), allergy or mucosal congestion, vigorous Valsalva maneuvers. Victims usually complain of pain and fullness of the ear which often causes divers to abort their dive. If they do not stop diving, their eardrum may rupture. Vertigo (spinning sensation), nausea or disorientation may develop. Inner ear barotrauma also can occur during descent with hearing loss, vertigo, hearing loss, incoordination & ringing in the ears (tinnitus).

Prevention & Treatment: Divers with vertigo or severe ear pain during descent should ascend in a controlled fashion. Treatment consists of bed rest, decongestants & antihistamines. Oral antibiotics are used for a ruptured ear drum. Surgery may be required for severe ear drum rupture or certain types of inner ear barotrauma.

NITROGEN NARCOSIS

Background:

- Nitrogen narcosis is due to breathing compressed air or oxygen/nitrogen mixtures during dives below 70-100 feet of salt water [fsw] (21-31 meters).
- Nitrogen narcosis is also known as rapture of the deep, the narcs, and inert gas narcosis.

Features: Nitrogen narcosis causes symptoms similar to alcohol intoxication with loss of coordination, disorientation, impaired, and loss of consciousness at increased depths (esp. > 300-350 feet salt water [fsw]).

Prevention & Treatment: Nitrogen narcosis can be prevented by avoiding depths > 100 fsw. Use of helium/oxygen mixtures can prevent nitrogen narcosis. Treatment consists of ascending to shallower depths.

OXYGEN TOXICITY

Background:

- Normal air is comprised of 21% oxygen
- A higher than normal inspired oxygen percent (> 21%) and higher than normal oxygen pressure (diving) can cause oxygen toxicity.
- Diving below 170 feet of salt water (fsw) can cause oxygen toxicity even with a normal inspired oxygen fraction.

Features: During diving, symptoms of oxygen toxicity can include muscle twitching, lightheadedness, loss of vision or hearing, confusion, and seizures.

Prevention & Treatment: Adherence to dive tables will prevent oxygen toxicity for recreational scuba divers. Use of low oxygen mixtures (e.g. 10%) at very deep depths (> 170 fsw), can prevent oxygen toxicity.

Encephalitis Overview

Encephalitis is an inflammation of the brain tissue. Viruses are the most common cause although bacterial, parasites, and fungi can also cause this disease. Mosquitoes, ticks, and mammals can carry the causative agents. In the United States herpes simplex, West Nile virus, cytomegalovirus, entoeroviruses, and togaviruses (eastern and western equine viruses) are most common. Those who are immunocompromised are at risk for these viruses and parasites (Toxoplasmosis) and bacteria (tuberculosis, Listeria).

Japanese Encephalitis (JE)

Background:

- The virus causing JE is transmitted by mosquitoes found in Asia and the Western Pacific including Southeast Asia, China, Japan, Korea, Eastern Russia, and India.
- Mosquitoes carrying the JE virus breed in wet areas including flooded fields and rice paddies.
- Mosquitoes transmit the virus to wading birds and pigs while travel to areas with pig farms increases the risk of this disease.
- The risk of acquiring JE is only 1 in one million for short term travelers to urban areas where JE is found. Most risk occurs in those spending a long time in endemic rural areas.

Features: Most who acquire the JE virus have no symptoms with less than 1% becoming ill. Those with symptoms become sick 5-15 days after exposure with fever, vomiting, and headache. An altered mental status, abnormal movements, weakness, or seizures (esp. in children) may occur. Death occurs in 30% of symptomatic victims.

Prevention and Treatment: Two vaccines are available for preventing JE. Both are only recommended for travelers who are visiting endemic rural regions, and are staying > 1 month during the transmission season (e.g. rainy season). The older JE-Vax can be given if older than 9 months while the newer IXIARO is only approved if ≥ 17 years old. (See page 10). General mosquito prevention measures will also decrease the risk of acquiring this disease (See page 63).

There is no specific treatment other than supportive care and treating complications (increased brain edema) as they arise.

FEVER Overview

Many diseases can cause fever during travel, at their destination and upon return home. Associated symptoms can aid in narrowing down the possible disorders causing fever. Pages 31, 35, 36, 39, 41 and 46 detail the most common cause of fever in visitors to travel clinics.

Select Travel Related Diseases Causing Fever & Illness[1]

Syndrome	Disease (Vector)
Isolated Fever *(many eventually develop symptoms listed below)*	• Malaria (mosquito), Dengue (mosquito) • Rickettsia, spotted fever (tick or mite) • Scrub typhus (mite) • Leptospirosis (water, soil, animal urine) • Typhoid fever (contaminated food, water) • Acute human immunodeficiency virus • East African trypanosomiasis (tsetse fly)
Fever & Bleeding or Bruising	• Meningococcemia (humans) • Leptospirosis (water, soil, animal urine) • Malaria (mosquito) • Viral hemorrhagic fever - Ebola, Marburg Yellow fever, Dengue (mosquito, tick, rodent)
Fever & Brain or Mental Status Involvement	• Bacterial, parasitic, viral meningitis and encephalitis (human-human, mosquito, ticks, other sources depending on type). • Rabies (mammals, and bats) • Poliomyelitis (contaminated water)
Fever & Cough or Shortness of Breath	• Influenza (humans, birds, swine), • Legionella (humans, esp. in water systems) • Histoplasmosis (airborne, cave, construction) • Coccidiomycosis (airborne, in soil) • Q fever/*Coxiella burnetti* (airborne via animals)
Diarrhea	• See pages 31, 35, 36, 39, 41 and 46.
Fever & Jaundice (yellow skin)	• Malaria (mosquito), hepatitis (A [fecal-oral], B [body fluids]), yellow fever (mosquito), Leptospirosis, Relapsing fever (ticks, lice)
Fever & Rash	• Dengue, Typhoid, Leishmaniasis, Brucellosis, Lyme disease, Rickettsia, bacterial skin infection & abscesses.

List is not all inclusive and other disorders can fit within categories[1]

Fever vs. Hyperthermia: A fever occurs when there is an increase in the body set point for normal temperatures due to viruses or bacteria. The thermoregulatory centers in the brain identify a new set point (> 37°C/98.6°F) as normal and the body will work to maintain this new temperature. While bacteria and viruses causing fever can be harmful, the fever itself is usually not harmful. Those with normal brains & normal thermoregulatory systems will benefit from the fever as it aids in fighting illness and they can control their temperature.

Hyperthermia occurs when the external environment or an external factor (cocaine, amphetamines) causes an increase in body's temperature. Mechanisms to normally lower and control the body's temperature become dysfunctional and may be unable to lower the temperature. Antipyretics (acetaminophen, paracetamol) do not work to bring down the body's temperature in this instance.

Risk factors for Heat illness (Hyperthermia)

• High humidity in addition to high ambient temperatures
• Lack of acclimatization
• Excess exertion
• Excess salt intake
• Advanced age and very young age
• Use of anti-hypertensives (esp. β blockers, diuretics)
• Use of medicines with anticholinergic properties (phenothiazines, benztropine, antidepressants, antihistamines)

Minor Heat Illness

Heat cramps occur after exertion & are related to drinking dilute fluids (not enough salt). They are associated with excess sweating during exertion. Mild cases can be treated by ingesting 0.1-0.2% salt solutions 2 to 4 ten grain salt tablets [56 to 112 mEq] or ¼ to ½ teaspoon (5-10 milliliters/ml) of salt in a quart of water (950 ml). *Heat edema* is the development of swollen feet and ankles in nonacclimatized travelers who have no underlying heart, liver, venous, or lymphatic disease. A diagnostic evaluation may be required to rule out thromboembolism (blood clots), or development of cardiac or other physiologic derangement in those at risk.

Heat exhaustion occurs from dehydration during heat stress. Symptoms include weakness, fatigue, headache, vomiting, and cramping. Unlike heat stroke, the temperature is usually < 40°C or 104°F and the mental status is usually normal. Left untreated, heat exhaustion can lead to heatstroke. Treatment consists of rest, a cool environment, and fluid replacement (oral if mild, IV if severe).

Heatstroke

Background:
- Heatstroke occurs when the body can no longer control or lower its temperature.
- Early in heatstroke, patients can sweat especially if exertion related. The ability to sweat can be lost as heatstroke progresses.

Features: Heatstroke victims usually have a temperature > 40.5°C (105°F) and altered brain function (confusion, coma, seizures). Sweating may or may not be present. Oral, skin, and axillary (armpit) are inaccurate for measuring core temperature in heatstroke. A core temperature (rectal, esophageal) is needed to accurately monitor temperatures. Heatstroke can be "classic" or "exertional". Classic heatstroke victims are older, have underlying disease, are on medicines that increase heatstroke risk (page 97) and do not sweat. Exertional heatstroke victims are younger, exercising, still sweating, may have low blood sugar, and are at risk for severe acid buildup with muscle breakdown, kidney failure, and bleeding disorders.

Prevention and Treatment: Acclimitization, proper hydration with balanced fluid/salt solutions and limiting exercise or exertion can prevent heat illness.

Treatment consists of removal from hot environment and immediate cooling. The preferred method is via evaporation and can be accomplished by applying tepid water to the victim (e.g. spray bottle) and fanning. Ice packs to high blood flow areas (e.g. groin, neck, and armpit) are also useful. The goal is to drop the temperature to 38-39°C (100.4-102.4°F) and not overshoot & make the victim hypothermic. Intravenous fluids, airway & blood pressure support, and management of complications are best accomplished in an intensive care unit setting. Acetaminophen (*Tylenol*) is ineffective, while aspirin and alcohol baths are harmful to heatstroke victims.

MALARIA

Background:

- Malaria is a parasite infecting human red blood cells that is transmitted through the bite of a female Anopheles mosquito and rarely through blood products.
- There are 4 types of malaria parasites (*Plasmodium falciparum*, P. *malariae, P. ovale,* and *P. vivax*) with *P. falciparum* causing the most severe disease and being most resistant to medications.
- Worldwide, there are > 300 million cases and > 3 million deaths due to malaria every year with the majority of deaths in children ≤ 5 years old and most cases occurring in sub-Saharan Africa.
- Endemic areas include Africa, Central & South America, Asia, the Caribbean, the Middle East & Eastern Europe with the highest risk in sub-Saharan Africa, New Guinea, the Solomon Islands, Vanatu, and intermediate risk in the Indian subcontinent and Haiti.
- Before traveling to any potentially endemic area, search the centers for disease control (CDC) website for detail regarding which medicines are required in specific countries to prevent malaria (wwwn.cdc.gov/travel/default.aspx).
- To adequately protect against malaria, traveler's must use protective clothing, treated mosquito netting at night, and medications before, during, and after a trip to an endemic area.

Features: Symptoms are due to this parasite infecting and causing the breakdown of red blood cells with release of parasites and toxins into the blood. Blood stream infection causes paroxysms of fever, while break down of red blood cells causes jaundice (yellow skin, eyes). Patients become dehydrated with sludging of blood in the brain (stroke), in the lung (respiratory failure), in the kidneys (renal failure) with muscle aches, headache, seizures or confusion, rigors, sweating, abdominal pain with an enlarged spleen or liver, diarrhea, and cough or respiratory difficulty. Depending upon which strain of malaria is contracted, symptoms may resolve without treatment (esp. *P. ovale*), persist for months and relapse, or result in death (esp. *P. falciparum*). Diagnosis usually takes place by direct examination of the blood using a specialized technique (thick and thin smear). This test may need to be repeated over a 24-36 hour period to detect parasites within the blood stream.

Prevention & Treatment: *Prevention*: Because there is no vaccine, personal protective measure are required to prevent the development of malaria. Since mosquitoes carrying malaria feed at night, most transmission of this disease occurs between dusk and dawn. Personal protection should include those listed below with special attention given to protection at night (Table: Malaria Protection).

Malaria Protection

Remain in well screened areas as much as possible.
Wear clothing and shoes/boots that cover most of the body.
Spray rooms at night with pyrethroid/pyrethrin flying insect spray and consider using mosquito coils or candles.
Use mosquito bed nets at night.
Treat bed nets with insecticides (permethrin spray, deltamethrin).
Use insect repellent with 30% DEET (N,N-diethyl-m-toluamide) on exposed skin for children > 2 months to 12 years old (American Academy of Pediatrics [AAP]) & 50% DEET if adult.
Infants ≤ 2 months old, use carrier draped with mosquito netting fitted tightly with elastic. DEET - not recommended by AAP.

Chemoprophylaxis is the use of medicine to prevent malaria. Medicines are started before travel, continued during the trip, and for a period of time after the trip. A 1-2 week trial up to a month before the trip can be tried so that time is present to try alternatives in case individuals are intolerant of a drug. Travel medicine consultants choose medications based upon whether drug resistant strains of malaria are present at the travel destination, the trip duration, and the traveler's age, medical history, current medications, allergies, and medicine side effects. See dosing, and drug detail, page 127-133.

Chloroquine Sensitive Malaria: Chloroquine (*Aralen*) is the drug of choice if no drug resistant malaria is present. This medication should be started 1-2 weeks before travel, taken on the same day (once per week) during travel, and continued for 4 weeks after leaving the malaria endemic area. Hydroxychloroquine (*Plaquenil*) is an alternative also used for regions with chloroquine sensitive malaria. Side effects for both medicines include itching, nausea, rash, headache, blurred vision, and insomnia. Taking either with meals may improve tolerability. If travelers cannot tolerate either medicine, atovaquone-proguanil (*Malarone*), doxycycline, or mefloquine (*Lariam*) are used. See drug detail, page 127-133.

Chloroquine Resistant Malaria: Most *P. falciparum* is resistant to chloroquine except in the Dominican Republic, Haiti, Central American west of the Panama Canal, and some areas of the Mid East. The following drugs are used for prophylaxis (see pg 127-133).
(1) Atovaquone-proguanil (*Malarone*) is started 1-2 days before travel, taken daily with food during travel, & 7 days after travel. Common side effects include abdomen pain, vomiting, and headache. It is not recommended in pregnancy, for infants < 5 kilograms (kg), or women breastfeeding infants < 5 kg or in severe kidney disease.
(2) Doxycycline is started 1-2 days before travel, taken daily during travel, and continued for 4 weeks after travel. Common side effects include gastrointestinal upset and rash or itching when exposed to sunlight). Doxycycline is not used in pregnancy or if < 8 years old.
(3) Mefloquine (*Lariam*) is started 1-2 weeks before travel, taken weekly during travel, and continued for 4 weeks after leaving the endemic area. Multiple neurologic (brain and mood) and gastrointestinal (abdominal) related side effects can occur. It should not be used if you have a history of psychosis, seizures, depression, or a cardiac conduction abnormality. Mefloquine resistance is increasing and is documented in Southeast Asia (Thailand, China, Myanmar, Cambodia, Laos & Vietnam). See drug detail page 133.
Terminal prophylaxis or Anti-relapse therapy: *P. vivax* and *P. ovale* can cause relapsing symptoms years after initial exposure since they can reside dormant within the liver. This therapy is only recommended for persons with prolonged exposure to malaria in endemic areas (e.g. missionaries, and Peace Corps volunteers). Primaquine, taken daily for 14 days after departure from an endemic area, is used for this purpose. Primaquine in not used if you have a G6PD enzyme deficiency or in pregnancy or during lactation unless the breast fed infant has a normal G6PD level.
Disease Treatment: Development of fever during travel or within months after travel to an endemic area requires prompt evaluation. The CDC recommends self treatment for travelers in remote areas who develop fever, chills, or other flu-like symptoms if no medical care is available. If not taking *Malarone* for prophylaxis, this medication can be taken for 3 days to treat symptoms. *Coartem* is another option for non-severe disase (page 127). Discuss presumptive self treatment regimens with your doctor prior to travel.

Punctures Caused by Marine Life[1]

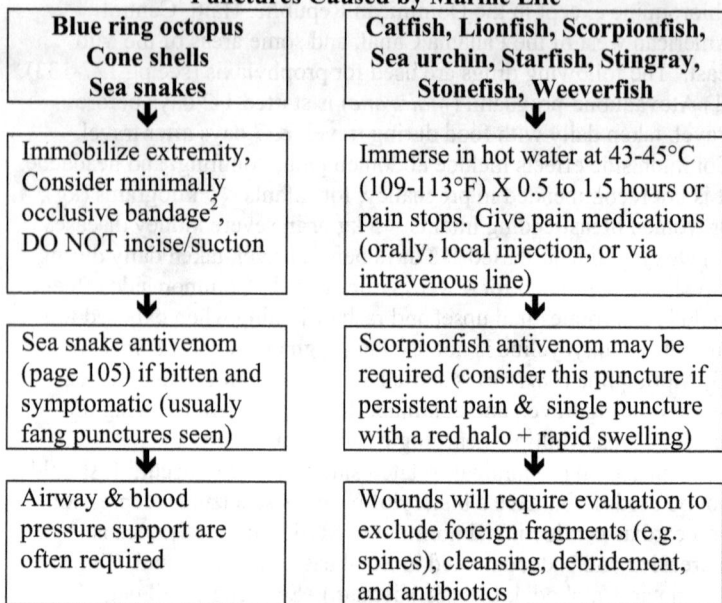

Blue ring octopus Cone shells Sea snakes	Catfish, Lionfish, Scorpionfish, Sea urchin, Starfish, Stingray, Stonefish, Weeverfish
Immobilize extremity, Consider minimally occlusive bandage[2], DO NOT incise/suction	Immerse in hot water at 43-45°C (109-113°F) X 0.5 to 1.5 hours or pain stops. Give pain medications (orally, local injection, or via intravenous line)
Sea snake antivenom (page 105) if bitten and symptomatic (usually fang punctures seen)	Scorpionfish antivenom may be required (consider this puncture if persistent pain & single puncture with a red halo + rapid swelling)
Airway & blood pressure support are often required	Wounds will require evaluation to exclude foreign fragments (e.g. spines), cleansing, debridement, and antibiotics

[1] Detail regarding most serious punctures is listed in following text.
[2] Apply a pressure bandage (pressure immobilize) from below the bite upwards as far as possible to compress lymphatics on the affected limb. Apply as tight as for an ankle sprain without affecting pulses. **CAUTION:** if too tight, this can increase tissue damage.

Blue Ring Octopus

Background: The blue ring octopus lives in waters off of Australia, New Zealand, New Guinea & Japan. It hides under rocks, or objects and shells in shallow water. This octopus is small and usually < 20 centimeters (8 inches). At rest, it is covered with brown & yellow bands. If excited, it darkens & blue circles or stripes appear.
Features: Most bites are from handling or picking up the octopus with few bites reported while it is in the water. Bites are painless punctures with numbness and aching of the extremity. Weakness occurs with paralysis of breathing muscles leading to death.
Prevention & Treatment: No octopi should be handled. Expect breathing difficulty and support respirations for up to 10-12 hours.

Catfish

Background: Catfish and stingray stings are the most common fish envenomations (venom injection). Catfish are found in muddy rivers, lakes, and beaches in tropical and subtropical salt and fresh water. Each catfish has 1 dorsal and 2 pectoral fin spines. Each spine has a stinging apparatus.

Features: Stinging occurs from handling or stepping on catfish spines. Wounds are extremely painful with tingling, numbness, bleeding, swelling, and cyanosis (blue or purple discoloration).

Prevention & Treatment: Do not handle catfish spines. Immediately wash away any existing venom with water. Then immerse the area in water at 43-45°C (109-113°F) for 30-90 minutes since heat destroys this venom. Remove spines or visible debris from wound. Wound exploration and Xrays, sonogram, or CT scan may be required to detect spines. Wounds need vigorous cleaning but not suturing or closure. Depending upon the local trauma, victim's health, and presence of foreign material, antibiotics may be required.

Cone shells

Background: Cone shells are cone shaped mollusks that feed on fish, worms, or other mollusks. Venomous species are found near southern Australia and in the Indo-Pacific waters. They burrow in the sand and coral during the daytime and emerge to eat at night. They feed by injecting venom with a tooth like apparatus.

Features: Stings from cone shells cause a painful puncture that may resemble a bee or wasp sting with burning or a sharp stinging sensation. Initial pain is followed by local ischemia (poor blood flow with pale, blue or purple skin), and numbness around the wound. Numbness and tingling may extend up the extremity and lead to muscular weakness (double vision, loss of reflexes, trouble swallowing or talking) including those muscles used to breathe.

Prevention & Treatment: Do not pick up a cone shell as it can inject venom in almost any direction near its shell. There is no antivenom available for treatment. Remove any debris (or radula/tooth) from the wound. Immersing the area in water at 43-45C (109-113F) may inactivate the venom. Pressure immobilization may be effective (see page 69). Respiratory & blood pressure support may be required.

Lionfish, Scorpionfish & Stonefish

Background: These fish belong to the same class and are found in almost all climates but are most common in tropical and subtropical regions. They dwell on the bottom in shallow water, bays, coral reefs, and rocky coastlines. All of these fish have 12-13 dorsal (back) spines. Envenomation usually occurs when fish and their spines are stepped on compressing the venom glands at the base of the spine and allowing venom to pass into the wound.

Features: Lionfish usually cause mild symptoms, while scorpionfish cause more severe, and stonefish cause life threatening symptoms. Stonefish stings cause immediate excruciating and incapacitating local pain. The wound itself may become numb with severe surrounding pain. Scorpionfish and lionfish cause intense but less severe pain. Puncture wounds are usually seen following stings. Tissue around the sting is often blue (cyanotic), purple, or pale. Rapid swelling, redness, & warmth occur. Stonefish venom can cause paralysis of skeletal muscles (stopping breathing), and heart muscle (cardiac arrest).

Prevention & Treatment: Divers should inspect the ground when settling on the bottom during a dive. Do not handle these species. Immerse the affected area in water at 43-45°C (109-113°F) for 30-90 minutes since heat destroys this venom and relieves pain. Remove any spines or visible debris from the wound. Wound exploration or radiologic imaging may be required to detect barb fragments. Wounds should be thoroughly cleansed but not be closed. Depending upon the amount of trauma, the victim's health status, and the presence of foreign material, antibiotics may be required. A stonefish antivenom is manufactured in Australia (Commonwealth Serum Laboratories/CSL). Poison centers residing in large cities near where envenomations occur are most likely to have access to this agent. In Australia contact the Venom Research Unit at the University of Melbourne (telephone # 61-3-934447753). It is usually given as an intramuscular injection. For 1-2 punctures, give 1 vial (2000 units) of antivenom, for 3-4 punctures give 2 vials & for > 4 punctures give 3 vials. Some experts recommend administration via slow intravenous infusion after diluting in 50-100 milliliters of saline.

Sea Snakes

Background: Most poisonous sea snakes are found in tropical or subtropical water in the Pacific and Indian Oceans. They are not found in the Atlantic, Caribbean, or Baja. Hawaii is the only state with sea snakes. **Features**: 80% of sea snake bites do NOT inject venom. Bites are relatively painless. Symptoms include anxiety, muscle pain, weakness, double vision, dilated pupils, and difficulty breathing. **Prevention & Treatment**: Pressure immobilize the extremity (See page 69). Incising or suctioning the wound does not remove significant venom. Administer antivenom (≤ 36 hours after bite) for symptomatic victims. The agent of choice is polyvalent sea snake antivenom (Commonwealth Serum Laboratories). If unavailable, tiger snake antivenom (related species) can be substituted. Contact local poison centers for availability.

Sea Urchins

Background: Sea urchins are globular to round spiny sea creatures. Their surface is covered with spines that contain venom and pincer like structures (pedicellariae) that also can inject venom. Punctures occur from stepping on or handling or touching.

Features: Stings are intensely painful. Initial burning evolves into local muscle aching, redness, and swelling. Spines may break off or leave behind a dark dye. If multiple spines are embedded, vomiting, tingling, paralysis, delirium & breathing difficulty may occur.

Prevention & Treatment: Immerse affected area in water at 43-45°C (109-113°F) for 30-90 minutes. Remove spines or debris from the wound. Wounds should be thoroughly cleaned & not closed.

Starfish

Background: The most venomous starfish, the crown-of-thorns starfish, is found on coral reefs in the tropics from the Red Sea, to the Indian & Pacific Oceans, and the Gulf of California off of Panama. This starfish has venom containing spines projecting from its surface.

Features: A sting from a spine causes severe pain, bleeding, and swelling. Multiple punctures can cause numbness, tingling, or muscle weakness. Delayed skin reactions can occur. Less toxic starfish can cause a localized irritant reaction with itching.

Prevention & Treatment: The spines of the crown-of-thorns are extremely sharp and can easily penetrate diving gloves. Treat in the same manner as sea urchins above.

Stingrays

Background: Along with catfish, stingray injuries are the most common marine envenomations (injury with venom). Stingrays live mostly in salt water although there are freshwater stingrays in some South American lakes and rivers. The stingray tail has 1 or more barbed stingers and 2 venom containing grooves. While the stingray's venom causes intense pain it is rarely deadly unless an important organ (e.g. heart or lung) is punctured from the trauma.

Features: Stingray injuries usually occur when a victim unknowingly steps on a stingray buried in sand or mud. The stingray flips up its tail often hitting, lacerating, and injecting venom into the victim's foot or leg. This can cause a gaping laceration with darkened, purple or blue edges. Pain is usually severe.

Prevention & Treatment: In areas with a high population of stingrays, walking in shallow water with a shuffling gait may prevent injury. After excluding life threatening injuries, immerse the affected area in water at 43-45°C (109-113°F) for 30-90 minutes since heat destroys this venom and relieves pain. Remove any spines or visible debris from the wound. Wound exploration, X-rays or ultrasonography may be required to detect barb fragments. Wounds should be thoroughly cleansed but not be closed. Depending upon the amount of local trauma, the victim's health status, and the presence of foreign material, antibiotics may be required.

Weeverfish

Background: Weeverfish are colorful fish living in the Atlantic Ocean and Mediterranean Sea. They burrow under the sand or mud. They are aggressive and will attack unprovoked.

Features: Stings from weeverfish spines are extremely painful causing local itching, swelling, tingling, and numbness. Their toxin can affect nerves and muscles causing weakness, paralysis, seizures, breathing difficulty and death.

Treatment: Immerse the affected area in water at 43-45°C (109-113°F) for 30-90 minutes since heat destroys this venom. Remove any spines or visible debris from the wound. Wound exploration or X-rays or ultrasonography may be required to detect barb fragments. Cleanse but do no close wounds. Depending on symptoms, airway and blood pressure support may be needed.

Rashes/Stings Caused by Marine Life
(blisters, hives, welts, tentacle prints)

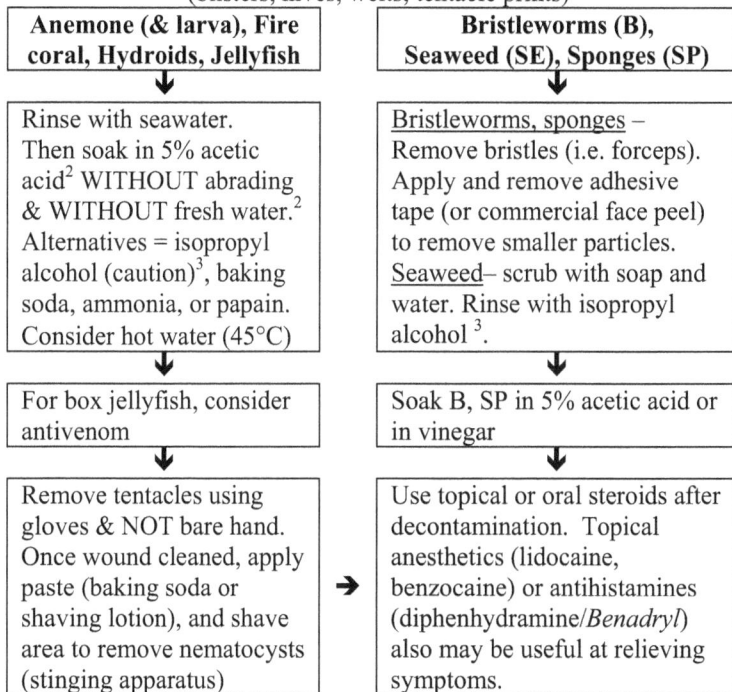

Anemone (& larva), Fire coral, Hydroids, Jellyfish	Bristleworms (B), Seaweed (SE), Sponges (SP)
↓	↓
Rinse with seawater. Then soak in 5% acetic acid[2] WITHOUT abrading & WITHOUT fresh water.[2] Alternatives = isopropyl alcohol (caution)[3], baking soda, ammonia, or papain. Consider hot water (45°C)	Bristleworms, sponges – Remove bristles (i.e. forceps). Apply and remove adhesive tape (or commercial face peel) to remove smaller particles. Seaweed– scrub with soap and water. Rinse with isopropyl alcohol [3].
↓	↓
For box jellyfish, consider antivenom	Soak B, SP in 5% acetic acid or in vinegar
↓	↓
Remove tentacles using gloves & NOT bare hand. Once wound cleaned, apply paste (baking soda or shaving lotion), and shave area to remove nematocysts (stinging apparatus) ➔	Use topical or oral steroids after decontamination. Topical anesthetics (lidocaine, benzocaine) or antihistamines (diphenhydramine/*Benadryl*) also may be useful at relieving symptoms.

[1] 5% acetic acid (vinegar) can increase pain in Portuguese Man-of-War stings and should not be used in this instance.
[2] Fresh water will cause the nematocysts (stinging apparatus) attached to the skin to fire and increase the pain.
[3] Isopropyl can cause nematocysts of some jellyfish species to discharge and should not be routinely used in this instance.

Anemone
Sea anemones are water dwelling flower like animals with a flexible cylindrical body and tentacles around a central mouth. The tentacles contain nematocysts (stinging apparatus) that sting. Red raised areas and blisters can occur. Soak the area in 5% acetic acid or vinegar. Do not use fresh water or alcohol.

Bristleworms

Bristleworms are elongated segmented worms often found under rocks and corals in tropical waters. Bites and stings cause inflammation, burning, numbness, and pain. The bristles penetrate the skin like cactus spines and are difficult to remove. Treatment consists of removing visible bristles. After drying the skin, apply a layer of adhesive tape to remove remaining small spines. Alternately, apply a facial peel or thin layer of rubber cement, then remove it. After bristle removal, pain relief can be accomplished by soaking in 5% acetic acid (vinegar), isopropyl alcohol (40-70%), or papain. Topical or oral steroids also may alleviate symptoms.

Hydroids & Fire Coral

Hydroids are fern like colonies occurring in clumps. Brushing against a hydroid causes burning or stinging pain with red raised areas. *Fire coral* has a bright yellow green and brown skeletal covering and appear in small brush like growths on rocks and true coral. It is often mistaken for seaweed. Remove any tentacles, ferns, or debris without using bare hands. Immobilize the extremity to prevent spread of venom. Soak the area in 5% acetic acid or vinegar. Do not use fresh water or alcohol.

Jellyfish

Background: Jellyfish are free floating animals with a main body, and dangling tentacles that have venom filled cells or nematocysts that inject toxins in response to stimulation. Jellyfish are usually found near the surface of the water during diminished light or after washing up on a beach. While most jellyfish are relatively innocuous, the box jelly fish (*Chironex fleckeri*) found primarily in Australia and the South Pacific can cause lethal injury.
Features: Most jellyfish cause intense stinging, itching, and red raised linear streaks on the skin. Occasionally, nausea, vomiting, abdominal pain, and muscle spasms occur. Box jellyfish tentacle prints form a classic cross-hatching or frosted appearance after applying aluminum salts. Box jellyfish can cause severe anaphylaxis (page 47), gastrointestinal symptoms (vomiting, diarrhea), headache, confusion, coma, paralysis, low blood pressure, breathing difficulty, abnormal heart rhythms and cardiac arrest.

Jellyfish continued ...

Irukandji syndrome is caused by an Australian species (Carukia barnesia) with minor stinging pain, muscle cramps, abdomen and chest pain, hypertension (high blood pressure), heart failure, and brain hemorrhage or swelling.

Prevention & Treatment: Jellyfish and free-floating, detached tentacles can sting for weeks after their death. For this reason, do not pick up any live or dead jellyfish. After excluding life threatening symptoms (shock or breathing difficulty), immediately decontaminate the victim. If no decontamination agents are available, rinse skin with seawater or saline to remove nematocysts. For **box jelly fish**, flood site with 5% acetic acid (vinegar) for 5-10 minutes before removing adherent tentacles. For other jellyfish decontaminate with vinegar, baking soda, or dilute ammonia for 30 minutes. Alternately, meat tenderizer (papain) can be applied for 15 minutes. DO NOT use isopropyl alcohol as this causes nematocyst to fire and sting. To remove remaining tentacles the area can be "fixed" with shaving cream or baking soda then shaving with a razor. Alternately, a paste of sand and seawater can be applied to the area and scraped with a shell or plastic credit card. Hot water (43-45°C/109-113°F) immersion will inactivate venom. Antivenom for **box jellyfish** envenomation is available from the Commonwealth Serum Laboratory of Melbourne Australia. Either 1 ampule is given intravenously or 3 ampules intramuscularly.

Portuguese Man-of-War

The Portuguese Man-of-War found in the Atlantic Ocean, Gulf of Mexico, the Pacific and Indian Oceans can kill. It is not a jellyfish. It is a colony of polyps. A blue gas filled float (bottle) floats above the surface of the water with a cluster of polyps from which hang tentacles that can be as long as 165 feet (50 meters). Stings from tentacle (nematocysts) can be painful leaving red welts. Remove tentacles (without bare hands) and rinse with salt water (not fresh water) to remove nematocysts. Hot water (43-45°C/109-113°F) will inactivate venom. DO NOT use 5% acetic acid (vinegar) as this can worsen the pain and is ineffective. This organism can cause life threatening anaphylactic symptoms. If any alteration in mental status, chest pain, or breathing difficulty occurs, seek medical care.

Seabather's eruption (sea lice, ocean itch)

Larvae of sea anemones and thimble jellyfish can find their way into bathing suits with resulting discharge of nematocyst (stinging apparatus). Freshwater (e.g. showering) will increase the itching and irritation. A red raised rash develops in covered areas, sparing exposed areas of skin. Treat by applying 5% acetic acid (or household vinegar) to affected areas with removal of swim suits before bathing. Topical or oral steroids may be used to treat severe eruptions. Make sure swim suits are washed or rinsed with 5% acetic acid or vinegar, then washed with soap or detergent before using.

Sea Cucumber

Sea cucumbers (sea slugs) are elongated sausage shaped creatures that live on the ocean/sea floor. Contact with the skin of a cucumber can cause skin irritation and severe eye inflammation. Apply 5% acetic acid, isopropyl alcohol, or papain to the skin. Irrigate the eyes with saline after applying a topical anesthetic (if available). Physicians may prescribe topical steroids for skin or eye irritation.

Seaweed Dermatitis

Seaweed dermatitis is due to contact with an irritating algae. The causative algae (Lyngbya majuscule) grows in clumps and looks like dark matted masses of hair or felt. This seaweed is black-green or olive-green, although it also grows in shades of gray, red, or yellow. Symptoms develop when small fragments of seaweed get caught between the swimsuit (or wet suit) and skin. This causes a red, burning, blistering rash in the swimsuit pattern.

Sponges

Sponges can cause a itchy, prickly, burning rash after the skin contacts the sponge's excrement. Soak in 5% acetic acid or vinegar until the pain is relieved. To remove sponge particles from the skin, apply adhesive tape to the area and peel it off. Then reapply acetic acid. Topical steroid creams or diphenhydramine (*Benadryl*) may alleviate persistent irritation and itching.

Meningococcal Disease

Background:

- The bacteria *Neisseria meningitidis* is an important cause of meningitis (inflammation of the fluid and lining of the brain) and meningococcemia (overwhelming bloodstream infection).
- This disease occurs in epidemic outbreaks around the world, endemically in sub-Saharan Africa, and during pilgrimages (esp. Hajj to Mecca, Saudi Arabia)
- This disease is easily spread by respiratory secretions and close contact increases the chance of acquiring the disease.
- During outbreaks up to 1/3 of individuals living in an area with disease will carry the bacteria in their naospharynx.

Features: The *Neisseria meningitidis* bacteria can cause two distinct clinical syndromes, meningitis or meningococcemia. Meningitis causes headache, fever, and a stiff neck and can lead to an altered mental status, confusion, and coma. Meningococcemia is an overwhelming blood stream bacterial infection and causes fever, shock, a red rash followed by bleeding under the skin, and respiratory failure with death occurring in as little as a few hours after onset. Both syndromes can occur separately or together.

Prevention & Treatment: Two vaccines are available for preventing the most common strains of this bacteria. Meningococcal conjugate (*Menactra*) vaccine (MCV4) is licensed for persons aged 2 to 55 years while *Menomune* vaccine (MPSV4) is used if over 55 years and may as young as 2 years if the MCV4 cannot be used. Administer if traveling to areas with a high risk of meningitis (hajj – Mecca, sub-Saharan Africa meningitis belt) if no contraindications exist. Vaccines must be given ≥ 10 days prior to travel.

Travelers suspected of developing meningitis or meningococcemia require hospitalization and intravenous antibiotics (penicillin G, ceftriaxone). They should be isolated until they are no longer infective.

Exposure to patients with Neisseria meningitidis disease requires prophylaxis with antibiotics. Adult regiments include rifampin 600 mg orally 2X/day for 2 days or ciprofloxacin 500 mg orally X 1 or ceftriaxone (*Rocephin*) 250 mg as intramuscular shot. Rifampin and ceftriaxone can be used in children.

SKIN DISORDERS

Determining the cause of a rash or skin disorder in a returning
traveler can be complex as there is significant overlap in the
appearance between serious and non-serious disorders.

Serious Travel Related Disease Causing Rash/SkinDiscoloration[1]

(See information regarding listed specific diseases within text)

Rash	Disease (Lists are NOT all inclusive)
Bites & Stings	See pages 51-74
Blisters (Bullae)	Allergic reactions and heat or chemical burns can cause blisters. Severe allergic reactions to many medicines can cause blistering & skin loss with dehydration & shock.
Blood or bruising or petechiae[2]	Meningococcemia, viral hemorrhagic fever, Rickettsia (spotted fever, scrub typhus, Q fever)
Fever & Exanthem *(widespread rash that is often red, and usually flat, or may be raised slightly above skin level [papular])*	< 14 days from exposure: malaria, dengue, typhoid fever, Rickettsia (spotted fever, scrub typhus, Q fever), Leptospirosis, viral hemorrhagic fever, trypanosomiasis, Histoplasmosis, coccidiomycosis, blastomycosis, borrelia. ≥ 14 days from exposure: Hepatitis, myiasis, amebiasis, trypanosomiasis, Lassa fever, Brucellosis, tuberculosis, HIV
Hives & Itching (Urticaria)	Allergic Reactions, When airway swelling, breathing difficulty or lightheadedness occur, allergy can be life threatening. See page 47
Jaundice (yellow skin)	Malaria, hepatitis, yellow fever, Leptospirosis, Relapsing fever (ticks, lice)
Red/painful	See skin infections, page 113
Target shaped[3]	Lyme disease, drug rash (Steven's Johnson)
Ulcers	Leishmaniasis, Trypanosomiasis, Fungi, *Mycobacterium ulcerans* (grass blades), multiple sexually transmitted diseases

[1] List is not all inclusive and many diseases listed can cause a wide
variety or rashes, and skin disorders (or may cause no rash)

[2] Petechiae – small areas of bleeding under skin.

[3] Bull's eye appearance, alternating, red & pale concentric circles.

Cutaneous Larval Migrans/CLM (Creeping Eruption)
Background:
- Cutaneous larval migrans is due to hookworm larva.
- 95% of victims acquire via walking barefoot on the beach.
- Infections occur in Africa, Caribbean, and South East Asia

Features: CLM causes an intense itching with a linear serpiginous (curving) rash that is 2-3 millimeters wide & grows 1-2 centimeters per day. Lesions are usually on the feet but can occur anywhere.

Prevention & Treatment: CLM can be avoided by not touching sand (or walking on beaches barefoot) in endemic areas. Adults can be treated with albendazole (*Albenza*) 200 milligrams twice per day X 3 days or ivermectin (*Stromectol*) 200 micrograms/kg orally X 1 dose or thiabendazole (*Mintezol*) 1.5 grams twice per day X 2 days.

Swimmer's itch
Background: Swimmer's itch is due to swimming in fresh water contaminated by schistosome larvae usually carried by aquatic birds.

Features: Red, itching, flat or raised areas occur soon after exposure and can last up to 2 weeks without treatment.

Prevention & Treatment: Swimmer's itch can be avoided by not swimming in infested lakes, toweling off after exiting water (removes larvae), swimming far from shore, and via application of water proof sunscreens. Treat with oral antihistamines (cetirizine/*Zyrtec*, diphenhydramine/*Benadryl*) and topical corticosteroids.

Skin Infections (bacterial) & Abscesses
Background: Methicillin resistant *Staphylococcus aureus* (MRSA) is the most common causes of skin infections and abscesses. MRSA abscesses are often mistakenly diagnosed as spider bites.

Features: Skin infections (cellulitis) can cause locally painful, reddened skin with an indistinct margin to the infection. Central to this area, skin abscesses (pockets of pus can develop). Systemic symptoms (fever, vomiting, and muscle aches) can occur.

Prevention & Treatment: Thoroughly cleanse skin lesions & wounds with soap & water. Do not pick at scabs, or pimples as this can introduce infection into the skin. Antibiotics effective against MRSA are used (*Septra, Bactrim*, clindamycin, linezolid/*Zyvox*)

UPPER RESPIRATORY INFECTIONS

Upper respiratory infections comprise a group of infections that include the common cold, laryngitis (inflammation of the voice box) or croup (in children), middle ear infections (otitis media), pharyngitis (throat infections), and sinusitis (sinus infections). Most of these infections begin as viral illness and only symptomatic treatment with over the counter cough medicines, antihistamines, or decongestants is needed. Antibiotics may be useful in a subset of bacterial pharyngitis cases (strep. throat – high fever, pus on tonsils, and anterior neck lymph nodes), and some but not all middle ear and sinus infections. Rare complications of disorders causing a sore throat include abscesses near the tonsils or posterior pharynx (throat) that lead to breathing or swallowing difficulty. In this instance, intravenous antibiotics and surgical drainage may be required.

LOWER RESPIRATORY INFECTIONS

The two primary lower respiratory tract infections include bronchitis (inflamed bronchial airways), and pneumonia (inflammation and infection of lung tissue).

Bronchitis

Background:
- Bronchitis refers to inflammation of the airways of the lungs.
- This disorder is usually due to viruses or allergy.
- Bronchitis is most common during the winter.

Features: _Acute bronchitis_ - A cough with sputum (mucous) production is the main symptom. Fever, runny nose, sore throat, centralized chest pain with coughing, and muscle aches are common. Wheezing can occur. Most are not short of breath.

Chronic bronchitis and emphysema are collectively referred to as chronic obstructive pulmonary disease (COPD). Chronic bronchitis is defined as a chronic productive cough for 3 months for 2 successive years. Chronic smoking and irritation from another source are common causes. Wheezing, chronic cough, recurrent respiratory infections, and shortness of breath are common.

Prevention & Treatment: If healthy, antibiotics are useless at improving symptoms. Those with chronic lung disease (e.g. chronic bronchitis, COPD) may benefit from antibiotics, steroids (prednisone), and inhaled wheezing medicines (e.g. albuterol)

Influenza/Influenzae – "The Flu"

Background:

- Influenza is very contagious virus with 10-40% of an exposed population developing the disease.
- Those < 1 year old, ≥ 65 years old, with underlying heart or lung disease, or with a weak immune system are most at risk.

Features: Symptoms often begin abruptly. Fever, sore throat, muscle pain & headaches are common. A mild cough that eventually becomes more severe is present. A secondary bacterial pneumonia may develop and may be life threatening.

Prevention & Treatment: Avoid sick contacts & wash hands with soap and water. Do not touch your eyes, nose or mouth. Vaccines are typically created against influenza A (H1N1, H3N2 strains) plus influenza B and prevent 60 to 90% of seasonal cases. All travelers should undergo vaccination prior to embarking on a trip (See page 9) Oseltamivir (*Tamiflu*) or zanamivir (*Relenza*) can shorten illness and limit complications if started within 48 hours of symptom onset. Both can prevent influenza if given within 2 days of exposure. Check the CDC website www.cdc.gov to determine if strains causing outbreaks have developed resistance to these drugs

Avian & Swine influenzae – Avian "Flu" & Swine "Flu"

Avian "flu" is a strain (H5N1) of the influenza virus. Waterfowl (ducks, geese) and poultry (chickens) are carriers. This strain can be transmitted to humans and cause severe disease with death in up to 30%. It is not easily spread between humans. Initial symptoms mimic influenza (the flu) with higher fever. Diarrhea is common. Unlike seasonal influenza, 70-100% of victims develop respiratory failure and require ICU care with breathing assistance. 42% develop heart failure & 1/3 kidney failure. **Swine flu is** a (H1N1) strain that carries genetic similarities to the virus that occurs in swine and in seasonal influenza. As of the spring of 2009, symptoms were mostly mild while death (<1%) and severe complications were uncommon although the very young were at higher risk than typical influenza.

Prevention & Treatment: Swine flu treatment is largely supportive with ~ 10% requiring hospital admission. Avian flu usually requires medical care in an intensive care unit with respiratory and blood pressure support. Oseltamivir (*Tamiflu*) and zanamivir (*Relenza*) may be helpful at treating patients with swine and avian influenza.

Pneumonia

Background:

- Pneumonia is an infection of lung tissue.
- Viruses, bacteria, parasites, and fungi can cause pneumonia.
- Like influenza, bacterial pneumonia is most common in the winter months.
- Advanced age, underlying heart or lung disease, weakened immune systems, alcohol and drug abuse increase the risk of complications from pneumonia (e.g. abscesses, fluid around lungs, blood stream infections) and unusual, difficult to treat organisms.

Features: Pneumonia symptoms can be mild mimicking bronchitis (cough, low grade fever, sore throat) or severe (altered mental status, low blood pressure, chest pain, short of breath, muscle aches, vomiting, diarrhea). Bacterial pneumonia typically causes a rapid onset of illness. A chest X-ray usually shows the infection within the lung tissue. Occasional cases are missed on X-ray and computerized tomography may reveal a hidden pneumonia.

Prevention & Treatment: Influenzae can predispose to bacterial pneumonia. Avoid sick contacts & wash hands. Do not touch your eyes, nose or mouth. Influenza vaccines prevent the types of pneumonia that occur following development of the "flu". Doctors may use a scoring system (CURB-65) to decide who may be safely discharged home. Typical oral antibiotics for healthy uncomplicated community acquired pneumonia patients include azithromycin, clarithromycin, moxifloxacin, levofloxacin, or doxycycline.

CURB-65		→	Total points	Admit or Discharge[4]
Confusion	1		0-1	Discharge
Uremia[1]	1		2	Admit
Respirations[2]	1		3	Admit
Blood pressure[3]	1		4	Admit
Age ≥ **65** years	1		5	Admit

[1] – Elevated BUN test (renal function), [2] Rate ≥ 30 breaths/minute, [3] BP ≤ 90/60 (either # below cutoff), [4] CURB-65 is not perfect at predicting who can go home and anyone with underlying illness, low BP, or other medical concerns may still require hospital admission.

Pneumonia - Legionella pneumonia, Legionnaires Disease
Background: Legionella is a bacteria that causes pneumonia, blood borne infection, or an influenza-like syndrome called Pontiac fever. Transmission occurs by aerosolization or aspiration of contaminated water. Legionella is found in whirlpools, spas (e.g. cruise ships), humidifiers, potable water systems (showers, faucets), cooling towers, and condensers. Risk factors include diabetes, cigarette use, steroid use, chronic heart or lung disease, kidney failure, or cancer.
Features: *Pontiac fever* is a mild infection due to Legionella bacteria causing an influenza-like disorder with fever muscle aches, and weakness. Pneumonia does not occur and victims improve within 3-5 days. *Legionnaire's disease* manifests with an acute fever, severe illness and pneumonia. Abdomen pain, vomiting, and diarrhea are common. Chest pain, bloody cough & altered mentation can occur.
Prevention & Treatment: Legionella infections can be prevented by maintenance of whirlpools, spas, and water systems. Treatment consists of antibiotics effective against this organism (azithromycin, levofloxacin, or moxifloxacin). If illness is severe, respiratory and blood pressure support in an intensive care unit may be required.
Pneumonia – Severe acute respiratory syndrome (SARS) is a viral life threatening pneumonia first described during major outbreaks, in China, Hong Kong, Singapore, and Canada. There is no treatment and up to 10% die. Symptoms include fever, cough and shortness of breath. This disease is highly contagious by airborne or other physical contact with droplets and prevention is accomplished via isolation of infected individuals. Treatment consists of supportive care. There are no proven effective anti-virals.
Pneumonia – Tuberculosis (TB) is a bacterial infection that can lead to chronic pneumonia. Prolonged contact with a contagious person in an enclosed environment is required for transmission. Rare cases have occurred in travelers directly exposed on prolonged air flights (> 8 hours). A TB skin test prior to traveling is required if prolonged TB exposure is expected. A skin test that changes from negative to positive 8-10 weeks after returning indicates a new infection. A vaccine (BCG) may be appropriate for individuals traveling to endemic areas for a prolonged time. If an infection develops, management by infectious disease experts with culture and sensitivity after a chest Xray will be needed.

Overview

There are at least 25 different organisms or diseases (e.g. HIV, gonorrhea, Chlamydia, hepatitis B & C, syphilis) that can be transmitted sexually. (Table) Many sexually transmitted infections (STIs) acquired during international travel are more likely to be resistant to standard antimicrobial drugs. While barrier contraceptives protect against STIs, they are not 100% effective.

Most Common Sexually Transmitted Infections (STIs)

Viruses	Bacteria	Fungi & Parasites
Hepatitis viruses	Chancroid	Histoplasmosis
HIV I, II	Chlamydia	Entamoeba histolytica
Herpes simplex	(urethritis, LGV)	"Jock itch" fungus
Papillomavirus	Gardnerella	(usually not an STI)
Cytomegalovirus	Granuloma inguinale	Giardia
Espstein Barr	Gonorrhea	Trichomonas vaginalis
Molluscum	Syphilis	Lice
contageosum	Shigella, Salmonella	Scabies

Travel STI Risk Reduction

The only way to reliably prevent an STI is abstinence or monogamous sex with a known uninfected partner.

Individuals with obvious sores, ulcers, or vesicles are more likely to transmit STIs

Use of drugs or alcohol inhibits decision making and can increase the risk of acquiring an STI

Sex acts that result in bleeding or that occur during menses increase the risk of transmitting viral STIs (HIV, hepatitis B & C)

Assume all commercial sex workers have multiple STIs

Prevention & Treatment

- Latex condoms reduce the risk of most (not all) STIs by only 50 to 80%. Latex condoms are better than animal membrane condoms.
- Prevention is preferred to treating STIs
- Travelers with one STI are at risk for other concurrent STIs
- Rapid diagnosis and treatment can reduce complications
- Diagnostic testing that includes cultures and sensitivity is required to guide therapy and assess resistance patterns
- Notify your treating physician or health care worker of your recent travel destinations to aid in making treatment decisions
- Notify partners to aid in their treatment and to prevent STI spread

Major Trauma

Major trauma including car accidents is the most common cause of traveler deaths in those under the age of 55 years. See Road and Car Safety section for details on decreasing the risk of these injuries.

    For victims of major trauma to the head, spine, or torso, brief stabilization and rapid transport to an appropriate hospital is the goal. At the scene of the accident, there are a few simple measures that may improve the outcome of trauma victims.

Bystander First Aid – Scene Tasks (if professionals unavailable)

Scene safety	Those providing first aid must make sure that they will not be harmed and that there are no ongoing threats to trauma victims (e.g. running vehicle, busy traffic, fluid/gas leaks, unsafe terrain, poor visibility, downed power lines)
Extrication *(Assume spine fracture is present)*	Awake, breathing trauma victims should not be moved. However, scene safety issues (e.g. fire) may require movement. In this instance, the victim's neck & back should be completely immobilized while moving them to a supine position, preferably with a board behind them.
Positioning Immobilization	Assume all major trauma victims have a spine (neck, back) injury and do not let them move. Keep in supine position.

Bystander First Aid (if professionals unavailable)
Victim Resuscitation for Non-Medical Personnel

Airway	If no air movement, lift jaw, do not move neck
Breathing	Rescue breaths are needed if not breathing.
Circulation (Stop bleeding)	Apply pressure to bleeding sites. Elevating legs is useless at improving circulatory status.
Disability	Check for responsiveness to talking, touching
Exposure (Hypothermia)	Look at patient head to toe for injuries and compress bleeding areas. Warm patient with blanket.
Rapid Transport	As soon as possible call for rapid transport to nearest facility able to care for trauma victims.

Abrasions & Cuts (Lacerations)

Abrasions are areas where the superficial layer of skin is scraped off. This injury occurs when skin and an object scrape against each other (e.g. road rash, carpet burn, rope burn). Bleeding is usually mild. This is in contrast to an avulsion where all layers of skin (i.e. a skin flap) are removed. For wounds where there is no suspicion of underlying bone, joint, or deep structure injury, treatment is aimed at preventing infection and scarring.

If available, anyone touching bodily fluids should wear gloves. Initial treatment consists of removing loose foreign material. This can be accomplished by rinsing with a forceful stream using water that is safe to drink. If no syringe is available, fill a plastic bag with water and puncture a pinhole in it. Squeeze the bag to create a forceful stream of water onto the wound. Next, scrub the abrasion to remove remaining debris and dead skin. Then, apply an antibiotic ointment and dressing. Re-clean the wound at least twice per day. Tetanus prophylaxis may be required. (See page 53)

Cuts or lacerations can be difficult to manage in a non-medical setting. If possible, exclude underlying injury to tendon, nerves, muscles, or bone and exclude foreign bodies (e.g. glass, debris). This often requires exploration after local anesthesia in a medical setting. Closing or suturing wounds is primarily accomplished to decrease scarring and stop bleeding. In general, closing a laceration or cut INCREASES the chance that it will become infected. For this reason, small cuts or lacerations are often not closed on the feet or on unimportant areas where scarring does not matter (e.g. scalp, trunk).

Caretakers should wear protective gloves. Control bleeding by applying direct pressure. Cleanse and irrigate the wound after removing debris as described for abrasions. Small (≤ 3 centimeter) wounds can be closed with glue (cyanoacrylate) by applying the glue over the closed approximated edges of the wound and holding in place for one minute. Keep these areas dry for 2-4 days. If medical "glue" is unavailable, Super or Krazy Glue may be used. For wounds left open, apply antibiotic ointment and a dressing. Wounds that are dirty also can be closed on a delayed basis after thorough cleansing and a short course of antibiotics. For clean wounds, suturing can be delayed 12-24 hours. Tetanus prophylaxis may be required.

Bones & Joints (Upper & Lower Extremities)

A fracture or broken bone is described as *closed* if the skin is intact and *open* if it pierces the skin. Open fractures require thorough cleansing ± surgery. Dislocations occur when bones within a joint become displaced. A Subluxation is a partial dislocation where the bone is still partially aligned with the joint. The most common joint dislocations involve the shoulders, fingers, knees, elbows, and wrists. Select fracture and dislocation complications that may require emergent treatment by medical professionals are listed.

Early Fracture & Dislocation Complications[1]

Injury	Features
Arterial injury	Cold and blue distant to fracture site. Absence of pulses. Severe pain distant to fracture site. After pressing toe or finger, pink color does not return within 2 seconds (capillary refill test).
Blood loss	Rapid swelling to extremity or visible blood loss for open fractures.
Compartment syndrome	Due to excess swelling of muscles within a closed space. Pain while passively moving muscle within compartment (most commonly below elbow or below knee). The extremity can become pale, with diminished pulses, limited movement affected muscles & tendons.
Contamination - Foreign body	Any cut or laceration near a fracture site should raise suspicion for an open fracture or foreign body greatly increasing the risk of infection.
Nerve trauma	Loss of sensation distant to fracture and inability to move beyond fracture site.
Tendon Injury	Inability to move specific muscle groups.

[1] List is not all inclusive as other immediate complications can occur.

Fracture & Dislocation First Aid

• Exclude life threatening injury – see Major Trauma, page 119
• Apply pressure to any active bleeding with sterile bandage
• Immobilize the area & the joint above and below the fracture if possible (rolls of newspaper or strips of wood can be used)
• Apply ice pack or ice wrapped in cloth to swollen areas
• If easily done, elevate the injured area above level of heart
• Have victim transported to nearest appropriate medical facility

URINARY TRACT INFECTIONS (UTIs)
& HONEYMOON CYSTITIS

Background:
- Several factors increase a traveler's risk of developing urinary infections (UTIs) including: delays in voiding, increased sexual activity, poor hydration, & less ability to practice good hygiene.
- Honeymoon cystitis is the term used to describe the increased incidence of UTIs in women while on vacation or honeymoon as a result of increased sexual activity.
- Women are more prone develop UTIs compared to men due to their shorter urethra (the tube from the bladder to the outside).
- Men with enlarged prostates or who are uncircumcised are at increased risk of urine infections.
- Sexually transmitted diseases can mimic the symptoms of UTI.

Features: Symptoms of a urinary tract infection (UTI) include painful or burning on urination, passage of frequent, small amounts of urine, blood in urine, and a feeling that the bladder will not empty. Left untreated, UTIs can cause kidney infection with fever, vomiting, back pain, and occasionally abdominal pain. Importantly, sexually transmitted disease (e.g. gonorrhea, Chlamydia, Trichomonas) can simulate or mimic urinary infections. Urethral or vaginal discharge may or may not accompany these infections.

Prevention & Treatment:
Measures to Prevent UTIs and Honeymoon Cystitis

Keep well hydrated
Do not delay emptying bladder (do not hold urine)
Urinate immediately after sex
Limit caffeine intake (prevents sensation of UTI but not UTI itself)
Consider D-mannose supplementation[1] (cranberry juice)
Phenazopyridine (*Pyridium, Azo*) relieves symptoms but does not cure urinary tract infections

[1] D-mannose is the substance in cranberry juice that stops bacteria from attaching to the wall of the bladder.

Antibiotics are used to treat UTIs. Options include ciprofloxacin, levofloxacin, trimethoprim-sulfamethoxazole (*Septra, Bactrim*), macrodantin and cephalosporins (cefixime, cephalexin). Healthy young women can be treated for 3-5 days. In most other instances, longer courses are required. (e.g. 7-10 days) Intravenous antibiotics are required for those who are immunocompromised or ill. Failure to respond to treatment may indicate bacteria causing the infection are resistant to medications, a urinary tract abnormality (e.g. kidney stone, enlarged prostate), or an alternate disease is causing symptoms (sexually transmitted disease, bladder irritation from pelvic or abdominal disease [e.g. ovarian cyst]).

Phenazopyridine (*Pyridium, Azo*) can relieve pain and burning within the urethra or bladder. This agent does not cure the infection.

Schistosomiasis

Background:

- Schistosomiasis is caused by a parasite that lives in freshwater snails in endemic tropical and subtropical areas including Africa, South America, the Caribbean, the Middle East, and Asia.
- Immature larvae enter the skin causing a rash before migrating to the lungs, the liver, and then the bowel or urinary tract.

Features: Initial skin penetration by larvae causes an itchy raised rash (urticaria) within hours. Within 2 weeks to 3 months delayed infection occurs (Katayama syndrome) with fever, weakness, muscle aches, abdomen pain, an itchy rash, and a cough with lung infection. These symptoms often resolve in a few weeks.

Chronic symptoms: Months to years after the initial infection, painful urination or blood in *urine* can develop. *Abdomen* pain, bloody diarrhea and liver inflammation can also develop. Less frequently, *lung* involvement can cause shortness of breath while involvement of the *nervous system* can cause seizures or an altered mental status or weakness.

Prevention and Treatment: Travelers can avoid this parasite by not swimming in fresh water and not using contaminated water to bath in endemic areas. No vaccine is available for prevention.

Praziquantel (*Biltricide*) is given at 20-25 milligrams per kilogram per dose X 3 doses over 1 day. Some experts recommend repeating the same dose in 1-2 months to kill developing worms.

YELLOW FEVER

Background:
- Yellow fever is a viral infection transmitted by mosquitoes.
- Infections can be clinically unapparent (up to 50% of cases) or life threatening.
- Most cases occur between 15° north and 10° degrees south of the equator with 90% of cases occurring in Africa and 10% of cases in South America (mostly January to March in forestry or agricultural workers).
- As of 2008, no yellow fever cases had been documented in Asia.

Features: Yellow fever develops 3-6 days following a mosquito bite. There are three phases of infection. (1) Initially, there is viremia (virus replication in blood stream) causing fever, headache, muscle and back pain, conjunctival injection (irritated white part of eyes), a relatively low heart rate for the degree of fever, abdomen pain and vomiting which last 3-4 days. (2) Over the next 1-2 days, symptoms remit. (3) A severe intoxication phase occurs in 15% of infected victims with liver inflammation (jaundice or yellow skin & eyes), kidney failure, an altered mental status, and shock. Bleeding from the nose, gastrointestinal tract, under the skin, gums and vagina can occur. Shock and death follow in 20-50% who reach this stage.

Prevention & Treatment: Mosquito precautions are important for preventing this disease when traveling to endemic areas. (page 63). A live vaccine is available and should be administered if traveling to endemic areas. The vaccine must be given at least 10 days before travel and immunity is conferred for at least 10 years. The vaccine is not recommended in infants < 6-9 months old, pregnant or nursing women, immunocompromised individuals (e.g. certain cancers, HIV, or on drugs that weaken the immune system), or those who are allergic to eggs or who are receiving other concurrent vaccine.

Treatment of yellow fever requires an intensive care unit setting and consists of blood pressure and respiratory support, blood products if needed, gastrointestinal bleeding prophylaxis (e.g. H2 antagonists), dialysis for renal failure, and management of complications as they develop. No antiviral medications are currently recommended for treating this disease.

Important Notice/Cautions Regarding Medications

Listed medications should only be taken under the direct supervision of a treating physician after a careful evaluation of each individual's age, pregnancy status, underlying illness, medical history, current medications, allergy history, and indications and contraindications for each medication to be taken. For **pediatric dosing, NEVER EXCEED** maximum adult dose listed for each medication.

Category	United States Food and Drug Administration Pregnancy Class of Medications:
A	Adequate well controlled studies have failed to show a risk to the fetus in the 1st trimester (1st 3 months) and there is no evidence of risk later (3 to 9 months)
B	Animal studies failed to demonstrate risk to the fetus and there are no well controlled studies in pregnancy women OR If animal studies have shown an adverse risk, well controlled studies in pregnancy women have shown no risk to the fetus in any trimester.
C	No adequate studies in pregnancy and animal studies have shown a harmful effect. Potential benefits of the drug may warrant its use despite the potential risk.
D	Human fetal risk has been shown although potential benefits may warrant use of the drug in select cases.
X	There is fetal risk and there are no indications for using these agents.

ABBREVIATIONS: g – grams, mg – milligrams, kg – kilogram, PO – give orally or by mouth, IM – intramuscular injection, X - times

acetaminophen (*Tylenol*)

Use: Pain and fever control. In general, acetaminophen will lower a fever by 2-3 degrees Fahrenheit for 4 to 6 hours.

Adult: 325 to 1,000 mg PO every 4 to 6 hours. Do not exceed 4 grams in a day. Rectal suppository is available.

Pediatric: 15 mg/kg PO every 4 hours. For those not taking any acetaminophen recently, some experts recommend a single 30 mg/kg loading dose, followed in 4 hours by 15 mg/kg. Do not exceed 4 grams in a day.

Pregnancy Class: B

Cautions: Do not take for a prolonged time, or if liver disease (especially alcoholics, or hepatitis).

acetazolamide (*Diamox*)
Use: Prophylaxis for acute mountain sickness, high altitudes
Adult: 125 to 250 milligrams 2 or 3 times per day beginning 1 to 2
days before ascent and 5 or more days after ascent.
Pediatric: Not established
Pregnancy Class: C
Cautions: Multiple adverse reactions are reported including ringing
in ears, vomiting, diarrhea, acid build-up, severe skin disorders.

albendazole (*Albenza*)
Use: cutaneous larval migrans (CLM), hookworms (H), pinworms
(P), roundworms ®.
Adult: CLM - 200 mg PO 2 X per day for 3 days;
H, P, R – 400 mg once
Pediatric: CLM – 7.5 mg/kg (maximum 200 mg dose) PO twice per
day X 3 days; H, P, R – 15 mg/kg once.
Pregnancy Class: C
Cautions: Gastrointestinal upset, vomiting, immune system
depression with low white blood cell count, headache, dizziness.

amoxicillin (*Amoxil*)
Use: Multiple infections esp. of throat, sinuses, ears, lungs, Lyme
disease, anthrax exposure (if proven susceptible to amoxicillin). This
drug is usually poorly effective vs. skin and urinary tract infections.
Adult: 250 - 500 mg PO 3 X per day or 875 mg PO 2 X per day. For
resistant infections up to 1 g 3 X per day can be used.
Pediatric: 40-90 mg/kg per day (divided so it is taken 3 X per day).
Pregnancy Class: B
Cautions: allergy penicillin class of antibiotics may also show similar
reaction to cephalosporin class of antibiotics.

amoxicillin-clavulanate (*Augmentin, Augmentin XR*)
Use: See amoxicillin, and used for cat or dog bite infections.
Adult: 250-500 PO 3 X per day or 875 mg PO 2 X per day. For
difficult to treat infections up to 2 g can be taken 2 X per day.
Pediatric: 40-90 mg/kg per day (divided so it is taken 2 X per day).
Pregnancy Class: B
Cautions: See amoxicillin

See Notices, Cautions, Pediatric Dosing, Abbreviations page 125.

artemether-lumefantrine (*Coartem*)
Use: Uncomplicated malaria
Adult: 4 tabs twice per day X 3 days. On day 1, give 2nd dose 8
hours after first dose. Peds: 1 tab (if 5-14 kg), 2 tabs (15-24 kg), 3
tabs (25-34 kg), 4 tabs ($\geq$ 35 kg); Pregnancy C; Cautions: multiple.

atovaquone (A)-proguanil (P) (*Malarone*)
Use: Malaria prophylaxis and treatment. Do not use as treatment if
already using *Malarone* for prophylaxis. Malarone is NOT approved
for prophylaxis of child if $\leq$ 11 kg or for treatment if $\leq$ 5 kg.
Adult: *Malaria prophylaxis* – 1 adult tablet (250mgA/100mgP) daily
start1-2 days pre-exposure, continue until 7 days after exposure.
Malaria treatment – 4 tabs daily X 3 days. Take with food or milk at
same time each day. If vomit within 1 hour of taking, repeat dose.
Pediatric: Pediatric tablets – (62.5 mg A/25 mg P). *Malaria
prophylaxis* – If weight 11-20 kg (1 peds tablet), if 21-30 kg (2 peds
tablets), if 31-40 kg (3 peds tablets) if > 40 kg use 1 adult tablet PO
every day starting 1-2 days pre-exposure until 7 days after exposure.
Malaria treatment – If weight 5-8 kg (1 peds tablet), if 9-10 kg (2
peds tables), if 11-20 kg (1 adult tablet), if 21-30 kg (2 adult tablets),
if 31-40 kg (3 adult tablets), and if > 40 kg (4 adult tablets). For
treatment, give dose daily X 3 days and take with food or milk at the
same time each day. If vomit 1st hour of take dose, repeat same dose.
Pregnancy Class: C; Cautions: Vomiting, diarrhea, headache, and
abdomen pain are common. Avoid tetracycline, metoclopramide
(*Reglan*), and rifampin when taking this medication.

azithromycin (*Zithromax*)
Use: Pneumonia, sinusitis, otitis media (ear infection), typhus, strep.
pharyngitis, traveler's diarrhea, Chlamydia.
Adult: *Diarrhea* – 1 g PO X 1 or 500 mg PO daily X 3 days.
Pneumonia: 500 mg PO X 1, then 250 mg PO X 3 days.
Pediatric: *Diarrhea* – 10 mg/kg PO (maximum 500 mg) per day X 3
days. *Pneumonia, otitis media* (ear infection) – 10 mg/kg PO on day
1, then 5 mg/kg PO X 4 days. Pregnancy Class: B
Cautions: Do not mix with other drugs that prolong the QT interval
on the electrocardiogram as rare life threatening heart rhythm
abnormalities can occur.
See Notices, Cautions, Pediatric Dosing, Abbreviations page 125.

benzyl alcohol (*Ulesfia*)
<u>Use</u>: Head lice <u>Dose</u>: 4-6 ounces (if 0-2 inch hair), 6-8 oz (2-4 inch), 8-12 oz (4-8 in.), 12-24 oz (8-16 in.), 24-32 oz (16-22 in.), 32-48 oz (> 22 in.) <u>Pregnancy Class</u>: B <u>Cautions</u>: Avoid if < 6 months old.

cephalexin (*Keflex*)
<u>Use</u>: Treatment of mild skin infections, strept. pharyngitis, respiratory infections and uncomplicated urinary tract infections.
<u>Adult</u>: 250-500 mg PO 4 X per day X 7-10 days.
<u>Pediatric</u>: 25-50 mg/kg/day (divided into 3 or 4 daily doses)
<u>Pregnancy Class</u>: B
<u>Cautions</u>: Allergy to this drug may occur if you are penicillin allergic.

cetirizine (*Zyrtec*)
<u>Use</u>: Itching, skin allergy, and allergic rhinitis (runny nose).
<u>Adult</u>: 5-10 mg per day.
<u>Pediatric</u>: If 6-23 months (2 mg daily), if 2-5 years old (2.5 mg daily or 2 X per day OR 5 mg per day), if ≥ 6 years old use adult dose.
<u>Pregnancy Class</u>: B
<u>Cautions</u>: Causes sleepiness, fatigue, and dry mouth.

chloroquine (*Aralen*)
<u>Use</u>: Malaria prophylaxis/treatment unless resistant malaria present.
<u>Adult</u>: *Malaria prophylaxis* – 500 mg PO each week starting 2 weeks pre-exposure and continued weekly on same day during and 4 weeks after exposure. *Malaria treatment* – 1st dose - 1 gram PO. 2nd dose – 500 mg PO 6- 8 hours after 1st dose, 3rd dose - 500 mg PO 24 hours after 2nd dose, 4th dose – 500 mg PO 24 hours after 3rd dose.
<u>Pediatric</u>: *Malaria prophylaxis* – 8.33 mg/kg (of chloroquine phosphate) each week starting 2 weeks pre-exposure and continued weekly during and 4 weeks after exposure. *Malaria treatment* – 1st dose – 16.7 mg/kg (of chloroquine phosphate). 2nd dose – 8.33 mg/kg PO 6- 8 hours after 1st dose, 3rd dose – 8.33 mg/kg PO 24 hours after 2nd dose, 4th dose – 8.33 mg/kg PO 24 hours after 3rd dose.
<u>Pregnancy Class</u>: C
<u>Cautions</u>: This drug can cause eye damage, decreased hearing, muscle weakness, seizures, psychosis, delirium, vomiting, diarrhea, and abdominal cramping. Multiple drug interactions occur.
See Notices, Cautions, Pediatric Dosing, Abbreviations page 125.

cimetidine (*Tagamet*)
Use: Skin allergic reactions, ulcers, gastritis.
Adult: *Skin* - 400 mg PO 2 X per day.
Pediatric: S*kin* - 10 mg/kg PO 2 X per day.
Pregnancy Class: B
Cautions: Multiple drug interactions exist.

ciprofloxacin (*Cipro, Cipro XR [XR-extended release]*)
Use: Animal bites, brucellosis, plague, marine infections, meningo-
coccal exposure, typhoid fever, traveler's diarrhea, urine infections.
Adult: Meningococcal exposure – 500 mg PO X 1, Most infections
250-500 mg PO twice per day OR (0.5-1 gram per day if XR used)
Pediatric: Only recommended if no alternatives & serious infection.
Pregnancy Class: C
Cautions: Can cause tendon damage and increased risk of tendon
rupture in addition to potential joint/growth plate injury in children.

clarithromycin (*Biaxin, Biaxin XL*)
Use: Pneumonia, sinusitis, otitis media (ear infection), typhus, strep.
pharyngitis, traveler's diarrhea, Chlamydia.
Adult: 250-500 mg PO 2 X per day OR 1 g of XL once per day.
Pediatric: 7.5 mg PO 2 X per day.
Pregnancy Class: C
Cautions: See azithromycin cautions.

clindamycin (*Cleocin*)
Use: Skin (including methicillin resistant Staphylococcus aureus) and
oral, and dental infections.
Adult: 150-450 mg PO 4 X per day.
Pediatric: 8-20 mg.kg/day (divided so it is given 3 or 4 X per day)
Pregnancy Class: B
Cautions: Prolonged use can cause *Clostridium difficile* colitis.

crotamiton (*Eurax*)
Use: Scabies, anti-itch.
Adult: Apply from chin down, reapply in 24 hours, wash of in 48
hours. Pediatric: not approved. Pregnancy Class: C
Cautions: Do not apply to eyes, mouth, nose, inflamed skin.

See Notices, Cautions, Pediatric Dosing, Abbreviations page 125.

dexamethasone (*Decadron*)

Use: Anti-inflammatory, anti-allergy, croup, laryngitis, acute mountain sickness (AMS), high altitude cerebral edema (HACE).

Adult: AMS - 4 mg PO every 6 hours, HACE – 8 mg PO, then 4 mg PO every 6 hours.

Pediatric: 0.15 – 0.5 mg/kg PO every 6 to 8 hours.

Pregnancy Class: C

Cautions: Use for more than 5-7 days can cause suppression of natural cortisol production.

dimenhydrinate (*Dramamine*)

Use: nausea, sea-sickness

Adult: 50-100 mg PO every 6 hours.

Pediatric: Do not use < 2 years old, 2-6 years (12.5-25 mg PO every 6-8 hours), 6-12 years (25-50 mg PO every 6-8 hours)

Pregnancy Class: B

Cautions: Causes sleepiness, fatigue, and dry mouth.

diphenhydramine (*Benadryl*)

Use: Anti-allergy, anti-itch, insomnia

Adult: 25-50 mg PO every 4 to 6 hours.

Pediatric: 5 mg/kg/day (divided into doses every 6 hours)

Pregnancy Class: B

Cautions: Causes sleepiness, fatigue, and dry mouth.

doxycycline (*Vibramycin*)

Use: animal bite (esp. cats), anthrax exposure, bubonic plague, brucellosis, bubonic plague, Chlamydia, cholera, Legionnaires, leptospirosis, Lyme disease, malaria, methicillin resistant Staph. aureus (MRSA), murine typhus, pelvic inflammatory disease, pneumonia, scrub typhus, traveler's diarrhea

Adult: 100 mg PO 2 X per day

Pediatric: if > 8 years old: 2.2 mg/kg/day (divided into 2 X per day)

Pregnancy Class: D

Cautions: Do not give if ≤ 8 years old or if possibly pregnant. Can cause rash if prolonged sun exposure during & after use. Do not take with antacids, vitamins, or milk products.

See Notices, Cautions, Pediatric Dosing, Abbreviations page 125.

eflornithine (*Vaniqa*) – drug used for melarsoprol refractory *Trypanosoma b. gambiense* sleeping sickness, given as infusion.

erythromycin (*Eryc, E-mycin, Ery-tab*)
Use: Campylobacter, respiratory infections, pneumonia, Legionnaires
Adult: 250-500 mg PO 4 X per day
Pediatric: 30-50 mg/kg/day divided so that it is given every 6 hours
Pregnancy Class: B
Cautions: Vomiting, diarrhea, and abdomen pain are common.

famotidine (*Pepcid*)
Use: Skin allergic reactions, ulcers, gastritis.
Adult: *Skin* - 20 mg PO 2 X per day
Pediatric: *Skin* - 0.5 mg/kg PO 2 X per day
Pregnancy Class: B
Cautions: Multiple drug interactions exist.

hydroxychloroquine (*Plaquenil*)
Use: Malaria suppression and treatment
Adult: *Malaria suppression* – 310 mg PO once per week on same day. *Malaria treatment* – 1st dose: 620 mg PO, 2nd dose: 310 mg PO, 6 hours after 1st dose, 3rd dose: 310 mg PO 18 hours after 2nd dose, 4th dose: 310 mg 24 hours after 3rd dose.
Pediatric: *Malaria suppression* – 5 mg/kg PO once per week on same day. *Malaria treatment* – 1st dose: 10 mg/kg PO, 2nd dose: 5 mg/kg PO, 6 hours after 1st dose, 3rd dose: 5 mg/kg PO 18 hours after 2nd dose, 4th dose: 5 mg/kg 24 hours after 3rd dose.
Pregnancy Class: C
Cautions: Dosing is based on hydroxychloroquine base & not sulfate. 310 mg of base = 400 mg of sulfate.

ibuprofen (*Motrin*)
Use: Anti-inflammatory, anti-pyretic (fever reduction), pain relief.
Adult: 400-800 PO 3 X per day.
Pediatric: 10 mg/kg PO 3 X per day. Not approved < 6 months.
Pregnancy Class: B (D in 3rd trimester – months 6 to 9 of pregnancy)
Cautions: Can cause gastritis, GI upset, and worsen kidney disease (esp. if dehydration). Not approved for use < 6 months old.
See Notices, Cautions, Pediatric Dosing, Abbreviations page 125.

ivermectin (*Stromectol*)
Use: cutaneous larval migrans, onchocerciasis, pediculosis (lice), scabies, strongyloides (roundworm)
Adult: 200 micrograms(mcg)/kg PO X 1 dose, except onchocerciasis - 150 mcg/kg PO every 6 to 12 months
Pediatric: Not recommended if weight < 15 kilograms.
Pregnancy Class: C
Cautions: Can cause adverse reactions after treating onchocerciasis due to death of organism.

levofloxacin (*Levaquin*)
Use: Legionnaires, respiratory infections, traveler's diarrhea, urinary infections
Adult: 250, 500, or 750 mg PO daily depending upon severity of infection.
Pediatric: Not approved for use
Pregnancy Class:C
Cautions: Can cause tendon damage and increased risk of tendon rupture in addition to potential joint/growth plate injury in children.

lindane (*Kwell*)
Use: Lice (pediculosis), scabies.
Adult/Pediatric (> 2 years): Apply lotion overnight and wash off in morning. For scalp, use shampoo and wash of in 10 minutes.
Pregnancy Class: C
Cautions: Do not use if seizures or if < 2 years old. Keep away from nose eyes and mouth.

linezolid (*Zyvox*)
Use: Methicillin resistant *Staphylococcus aureus* – usually causing skin infection & abscesses although other body sites can be infected.
Adult: Skin – 600 mg PO 2 X per day.
Pediatric: 10 mg/kg PO 3 X per day.
Pregnancy Class: C
Cautions: Uncommon lowering of platelet count, rare nerve and visual side effects.

See Notices, Cautions, Pediatric Dosing, Abbreviations page 125.

meclizine (*Antivert*)
Use: motion sickness, vertigo
Adult: 25-50 mg PO pre-travel, then daily for motion sickness OR 25 mg PO 4 X per day for vertigo.
Pediatric: Not approved
Pregnancy Class: B
Cautions: Causes sleepiness, fatigue, and dry mouth.

mefloquine (*Lariam*)
Use: Malaria prophylaxis and treatment and chloroquine resistance
Adult: *Malaria prophylaxis* – 250 mg PO starting 1 week pre-travel and continuing weekly until 4 weeks after travel. *Malaria treatment* – 1.25 grams X 1. Some experts split dose into initial 750 mg, followed by 500 mg 12 hours later. Take on full stomach.
Pediatric: Do not use if < 5 kg or < 3 months old (some experts do not use if < 6 months old). *Malaria prophylaxis* – 5 mg/kg PO starting 1 week pre-travel and continuing weekly until 4 weeks after travel. *Malaria treatment* – 10 to 12.5 mg/kg taken 8 hours apart. Take on full stomach. If vomiting occurs < 30 minutes from taking medicine, repeat the entire dose. If vomiting occurs 30-60 minutes after administering, repeat ½ of the dose.
Pregnancy Class: C
Cautions: A second drug may be required if *P. ovale* or *P. malariae* is the causative parasite. Do NOT take this drug if seizures, psychiatric illness, heart rhythm abnormalities, or taking any other drug that can prolong the QT interval (electrocardiogram/ECG). This drug can cause drowsiness, lightheadedness, psychiatric symptoms, and gastrointestinal symptoms (vomiting, and pain) in addition to multiple other side effects.

melatonin
Use: Treatment of jet lag.
Adult: 2 to 5 mg PO at bedtime X 2 to 4 days.
Pediatric: Not recommended for jet lag in children.
Pregnancy Class: Not recommended.
Cautions: Production and manufacture is not regulated so dosing, purity, and impurities can be a problem.

See Notices, Cautions, Pediatric Dosing, Abbreviations page 125.

metronidazole (*Flagyl*)
Use: Certain gastrointestinal, gynecologic, and parasitic infections
(e.g. amoeba, Giardia)
Adult: *Amebic dysentery* – 750 mg PO 3 X per day X 10 days;
Giardia – 250 mg PO 3 X per day X 5 days
Pediatric: *Amebic dysentery* – 12 - 16.7 mg/kg 3 X per day X 10
days; *Giardia* – 5 mg/kg PO 3 X per day X 5-7 days
Pregnancy Class: B
Cautions: Gastrointestinal upset is common. Uncommon serious side
effects include seizures, and numbness, tingling of an extremity. Do
not take alcohol while taking this drug.

moxifloxacin (*Avelox*)
Use: Legionnaires, Respiratory tract (pneumonia, sinus) infections
Adult: 400 mg PO once per day X 5-10 days.
Pediatric: Not approved for children.
Pregnancy Class:C
Cautions: See levofloxacin cautions.

nifedipine (*Procardia XL, Adalat XL*)
Use: A blood pressure pill used by some experts to prevent and treat
high altitude pulmonary edema (HAPE)
Adult: HAPE Treatment or Prevention – 20 to 30 mg PO of
sustained release pill every 12 hours.
Pediatric: Not approved, some experts use for blood pressure control.
Pregnancy Class: C
Cautions: Can cause a drop in blood pressure.

nifurtimox (*Lampit*) – specialized drug for treating Chagas disease
only available from the centers for disease control.

nitrofurantoin (*Furadantin, Macrobid, Macrodantin*)
Use: Urine infections
Adult: *Macrobid dose* – 100 mg PO twice per day
Pediatric: Macrodantin dose (not *Macrobid*) – 5-7 mg/kg/day
(divided into 4 doses per day)
Pregnancy Class: B
Cautions: Do not use if G6PD deficiency or < 1 month old.

See Notices, Cautions, Pediatric Dosing, Abbreviations page 125.

ondansetron (*Zofran*)
<u>Use</u>: Nausea or vomiting.
<u>Adult</u>: 4 to 8 mg PO every 8 hours.
<u>Pediatric</u>: If weight 8-15 kg (2 mg), if weight 15-30kg (4 mg), and if weight > 30 kg (4 to 8 mg) every 8 hours.
<u>Pregnancy Class</u>: B
<u>Cautions</u>: Can worsen diarrhea.

paracetamol (see acetaminophen)

permethrin (*Elimite, Nix*)
<u>Use</u>: Lice (pediculosis), scabies
<u>Adult/Pediatric</u>: Apply lotion overnight and wash off in morning. For scalp, use shampoo and wash of in 10 minutes.
<u>Pregnancy Class</u>: C
<u>Cautions</u>: Keep away from nose, eyes, mouth and

phenazopyridine (*Pyridium, Azo*)
<u>Use</u>: Dysuria (burning with urination)
<u>Adult</u>: 200 mg PO 3 X per day X 2 days.
<u>Pediatric</u>: ≥ 6 years old – 4 mg/kg PO every 8 hours X 2 days.
<u>Pregnancy Class</u>: B
<u>Cautions</u>: Turns urine orange/red and can stain contact lenses.

praziquantel (*Biltricide*)
<u>Use</u>: Schistosomiasis (Sch), liver flukes, neurocystocercosis (not approved), tape worms
<u>Adult</u>: Sch – 20 mg/kg PO every 4 to 6 hours X 3 doses.
<u>Pediatric</u>: Sch - 20 mg/kg PO every 4 to 6 hours X 3 doses.
<u>Pregnancy Class</u>: B
<u>Cautions</u>: Multiple side effects and drug interactions

prednisone/prednisolone (*Deltasone, Orapred, Pediapred*)
<u>Use</u>: Allergic reactions, asthma, anaphylaxis.
<u>Adult</u>: 40 to 60 mg per day up to 1 week.
<u>Pediatric</u>: 1 to 2 mg/kg per day up to 1 week.
<u>Pregnancy Class</u>: C
<u>Cautions</u>: If taken > 1 week, suppresses internal cortisol production.

See Notices, Cautions, Pediatric Dosing, Abbreviations page 125.

primaquine
Use: Relapse of malaria prevention for P. vivax and P. ovale.
Adult: 30 mg PO of base daily X 14 days
Pediatric: Not approved although some experts may prescribe 0.5 mg/kg PO daily for 14 days.
Pregnancy Class: X highly unsafe, do not use
Cautions: A normal G6PD level must be documented prior to use. Can cause breakdown of blood cells if G6PD deficiency. Avoid if lupus, rheumatoid arthritis, or use of immune suppressants.

promethazine (*Phenergan*)
Use: nausea, vomiting, motion sickness
Adult: *Nausea/vomiting* - 12.5 to 25 mg PO or via rectal suppository every 4-6 hours. *Motion sickness* – 25 mg PO 2 X per day.
Pediatric: Never use if ≤ 2 years old. *Nausea/vomiting* – 0.25 to 1 mg/kg mg PO or via rectal suppository every 4-6 hours. *Motion sickness* – 0.5 mg/kg PO 2 X per day with 1st dose 30-60 minutes pretravel.
Pregnancy Class: C
Cautions: This drug can mask serious illness in young children so never use or use sparingly if 2-5 years, and never use if ≤ 2 years old.

pyrimethamine-sulfadoxine (*Fansidar*)
The US Center for Disease Control does not recommend use of this agent due to increasing resistance and severe life threatening skin & blood disorders, and infections that can occur with its use.

rifampin (*Rifadin*)
Use: meningococcal exposure (not treatment), scrub typhus, tuberculosis (part of multi-drug regimen), murine typhus, as 2nd agent in methicillin resistant *Staph. aureus*, as 2nd agent in brucellosis.
Adult: *Meningitis exposure* - 600 mg PO every 12 hours X 4 doses. Otherwise, 300-600 mg PO every 12 hours.
Pediatric: *Meningitis exposure* – If < 1 month: 5 mg/kg PO every 12 hours X 2 days, if > 1 month, 10 mg/kg PO every 12 hours X 2 days.
Pregnancy Class: C
Cautions: Take on an empty stomach.

See Notices, Cautions, Pediatric Dosing, Abbreviations page 125.

rifaximin (*Xifaxan*)
Use: Traveler's diarrhea
Adult: 200 mg PO 3 X per day X 3 days.
Pediatric: Not approved in children < 12 years old.
Pregnancy Class: C
Cautions: Gastrointestinal pain, gas, and nausea are common

scopolamine (*Transderm-Scop, Scopace*)
Use: Prevention and treatment of motion sickness.
Adult: 0.4 to 0.8 mg PO 1 hour pre-travel and every 8 hours as needed OR apply 1 disc behind ear 4 hours pre-travel and every 3 days as needed.
Pediatric: Not approved for use in children.
Pregnancy Class: C
Cautions: Can cause blurred vision, urine retention, decreased sweating, dry lips and mouth, and drowsiness.

sildenafil (*Viagra*)
Use: This drug is not approved for use in high altitude pulmonary edema (HAPE) however, some experts use for this purpose.
Adult: HAPE prevention - 50 mg PO every 8 hours. Dosing for treatment of HAPE is not determined.
Pediatric: Not approved in children.
Pregnancy Class: B
Cautions: Do not take if also taking nitrates. Can cause sudden drop in blood pressure, or sudden vision loss, or painful prolonged erection resulting in damage to penis.

tadalafil (*Cialis*)
Use: This drug is not approved for use in high altitude pulmonary edema (HAPE) however, some experts use for this purpose.
Adult: HAPE prevention - 10 mg PO every 12 hours. Dosing for treatment of HAPE is not determined.
Pediatric: Not approved in children.
Pregnancy Class: B
Cautions: Do not take if also taking nitrates. Can cause sudden drop in blood pressure, or sudden vision loss, or painful prolonged erection resulting in damage to penis.

See Notices, Cautions, Pediatric Dosing, Abbreviations page 125.

tetracycline
Use: animal bite (esp. cats), anthrax exposure, bubonic plague, brucellosis, bubonic plague, Chlamydia, cholera, Legionnaires, leptospirosis, Lyme disease, malaria, methicillin resistant Staph. aureus (MRSA), murine typhus, pelvic inflammatory disease, pneumonia, scrub typhus, traveler's diarrhea
Adult: 250-500 mg PO 4 x per day
Pediatric: if > 8 years old: 25-50 mg/kg/day (divided into 4 doses per day)
Pregnancy Class: D
Cautions: Do not give if ≤ 8 years old or if possibly pregnant. Tetracycline can cause a rash if prolonged sun exposure during & after use. Do not take with antacids, vitamins, or milk products.

thiabendazole (*Mintezol*)
Use: Cutaneous larval migrans (CLM), Strongyloides, visceral larval migrans (VLM), tungiasis; as 2nd line agent in hookworms, roundworms, pinworms, and whipworms
Adult: 22 mg/kg PO 2 X per day (maximum - 1.5 gram per dose). 2 day treatment if: CLM, Strongyloides, roundworms, pinworms, hookworms. Trichinosis requires up to 4 days and VLM requires 7 days of treatment with same dose
Pediatric: If weight > 13.5 kg: 22 mg/kg PO 2 X per day (maximum - 1.5 grams per dose). Treat for same duration as per adult regimens above.
Pregnancy Class: C
Cautions: Not approved if weight < 13.5 kg. Multiple side effects.

tinidazole (*Tindamax*)
Use: Amebiasis, giardia, trichomonas, vaginosis
Adult: Amoeba (not liver abscess) – 2 g PO daily X 3 days; giardia, trichomonas – 2 g PO X 1; vaginosis – 2 g PO X 2 days.
Pediatric: Amoeba (not liver abscess) – 50 mg/kg PO daily X 3 days; giardia, – 50 mg/kg PO X 1 dose
Pregnancy Class: C
Cautions: Do not use ≤ 3 years old. Further treatment for amoeba may be required.

See Notices, Cautions, Pediatric Dosing, Abbreviations page 125.

trimethoprim-sulfamethoxazole (*Bactrim, Septra*)
<u>Use</u>: bronchitis in adults, pediculosis (lice), skin infection (including methicillin resistant *Staphylococcus aureus*/MRSA), traveler's diarrhea (TD), urine infections (UTI). DS = double strength.
<u>Adult</u>: 1 *Bactrim DS* or *Septra DS* PO 2 X per day. <u>Treatment duration</u>: Lice – (3 days and repeat in 1 week), MRSA (7-14 days), TD (5 days), UTI (uncomplicated 3 to 5 days, complicated, older, or underlying disease – 10-14 days; urine pathogens are becoming increasingly resistant to this antibiotic)
<u>Pediatric</u>: 5 milliliters (one teaspoon)/10 kg PO every 12 hours. (Maximum dose = 20 ml every 12 hours). Treatment duration, see adult regimens above.
<u>Pregnancy Class</u>: C
<u>Cautions</u>: Do not use if < 2 months old.

zolpidem (*Ambien*)
<u>Use</u>: Jet lag treatment.
<u>Adult</u>: 10 mg PO during flights eastward and continued for 4 nights.
<u>Pediatric</u>: Not approved in children.
<u>Pregnancy Class</u>: C
<u>Cautions</u>: Multiple drug interactions and side effects. Zolpidem may cause drowsiness the day after using.

See Notices, Cautions, Pediatric Dosing, Abbreviations page 125.

Index 147

www.ingramcontent.com/pod-product-compliance
Lightning Source LLC
Chambersburg PA
CBHW071337290326
41933CB00039B/1295